Exploring End of Life Experience

The groundbreaking contribution made by this unique book draws on the experiences recorded by five people who are facing death – Jenny Diski, Philip Gould, Christopher Hitchens, Michael Mayne and Cory Taylor.

Analysing the key themes that emerge from a psychodynamic perspective, the book describes how the memoirists respond to the first shock of receiving a terminal diagnosis, how they meet the challenge of continuing an active life when the illusion of an open-ended future has gone, and finally, how they struggle with accepting death as it overtakes them. The author argues that the ability to accept personal death is the key to resolving the paradox of our need to survive at all costs, while at the same time, however much we might deny it, we know that we must die. In a society where death and dying occur largely out of sight, this book provides information about what it is like to die – physically, psychologically and emotionally – and invites us to think about coming to terms with death.

Exploring End of Life Experience is an important contribution to the interdisciplinary literature on death and dying, relevant to scholars and practitioners in medicine, nursing, psychology, and the wider medical humanities.

Dr Helen Besemeres is a retired psychoanalyst and family therapist, with a PhD in Education from Monash University, Melbourne.

Routledge Key Themes in Health and Society

Available titles include:

Older Citizens and End-of-Life Care
Social work practice strategies for adults in later life
Malcolm Payne

Digital Technologies and Generational Identity
ICT Usage Across the Life Course
Sakari Taipale, Terhi-Anna Wilksa and Chris Gilleard

Partiality and Justice in Nursing Care
Marita Nordhaug

Loss, Dying and Bereavement in the Criminal Justice System
Edited by Sue Read, Sotirios Santatzoglou and Anthony Wrigley

Professional Identity in the Caring Professions
Meaning, Measurement and Mastery
Edited by Roger Ellis and Elaine Hogard

Trade Union Strategies and Healthcare Marketization
Jennie Auffenberg

Leadership at the Intersection of Gender and Race in Healthcare and Science
Case Studies and Tools
Edited by Danielle Laraque-Arena, Lauren Germain, Virginia Young and Rivers Laraque-Ho

Exploring End of Life Experience
Facing Death
Dr Helen Besemeres

https://www.routledge.com/Routledge-Key-Themes-in-Health-and-Society/book-series/RKTHS

Exploring End of Life Experience

Facing Death

Dr Helen Besemeres

Routledge
Taylor & Francis Group
LONDON AND NEW YORK

First published 2024
by Routledge
4 Park Square, Milton Park, Abingdon, Oxon OX14 4RN

and by Routledge
605 Third Avenue, New York, NY 10158

Routledge is an imprint of the Taylor & Francis Group, an informa business

British Library Cataloguing-in-Publication Data
A catalogue record for this book is available from the British Library

Library of Congress Cataloging-in-Publication Data
Names: Besemeres, Helen, author.
Title: Exploring end of life experience: facing death /
Dr. Helen Besemeres.
Description: Abingdon, Oxon; New York, NY : Routledge, 2024. |
Includes bibliographical references and index.
Identifiers: LCCN 2023019538 | ISBN 9781032490847 (hardback) |
ISBN 9781032494128 (paperback) | ISBN 9781003392088 (ebook)
Subjects: LCSH: Death—Psychological aspects. | Death.
Classification: LCC BF789.D4 B477 2024 |
DDC 155.9/37—dc23/eng/20230707
LC record available at https://lccn.loc.gov/2023019538

ISBN: 978-1-032-49084-7 (hbk)
ISBN: 978-1-032-49412-8 (pbk)
ISBN: 978-1-003-39208-8 (ebk)

DOI: 10.4324/9781003392088

Typeset in Sabon
by codeMantra

Contents

Acknowledgements

To the following people and organisations:

Dr Jillian Brown
Professor Ken Cruickshank
Mrs Alison Mayne, and Publishers, Darton, Longman & Todd Ltd
The Baroness Gail Rebuck DBE, on behalf of Philip Gould
The estate holders for Jenny Diski, and Bloomsbury Publishing Plc

Most of all, I am indebted to my memoirists, Jenny Diski, Philip Gould, Christopher Hitchens, Michael Mayne, and Cory Taylor

I wish to express my heartfelt thanks to each of you for your generosity of spirit in supporting the commitment I make in this book to better understand and deepen our experience of facing death.

Acronyms

ABC	Australian Broadcasting Commission
ABS	Australian Bureau of Statistics
ACP	Advance Care Planning or Advance Care Plan(s)
AIHW	Australian Institute of Health and Welfare
AMA	Australian Medical Association
BMJ	*British Medical Journal*
CASPD	Commonwealth of Australia, Social Policy Division
CG	Commonwealth Government
CGDH	Commonwealth Government Department of Health
CPR	Cardiopulmonary resuscitation
ER	Emergency Room
GP	General Practitioner
ICU	Intensive Care Unit
MJA	*Medical Journal of Australia*
MSc	Master of Science
NHS	National Health Service (United Kingdom)
PCA	Palliative Care Australia
PVLC	Parliament of Victoria, Legislative Council
RACF	Residential aged care facility
RACGP	Royal Australian College of General Practitioners
RACP	Royal Australian College of Physicians
RN	Radio National
SMH	Sydney Morning Herald
VDHHS	Victorian Department of Health & Human Services
UK	United Kingdom
US or USA	United States, or United States of America
WHO	World Health Organisation

1 Death

An introduction

Part I. Facing death: The author's memoir

The alarm clock shrilled: it was seven o'clock, and time to get up. I swung my legs over the side of the bed as usual, stood up – and fell over. "Let's try that again", I advised myself, but again, apparently unable to keep my balance, I fell sideways against the wall. At this stage puzzled more than worried, I assessed my situation. I was staying in a hotel in Lowestoft in Suffolk, England, seventeen thousand kilometres from my home in Melbourne, and four hours' drive from my temporary home and child care workplace in London. I knew no one in Lowestoft, and I had a full day's work booked up vetting prospective foster parents. A fit twenty-nine-year-old, I had suddenly found myself unable to stand up without falling sideways. It was 1967, and mobile phones did not yet exist; in any case, my office colleagues would probably still be asleep. I decided that I had to cancel my appointments and somehow, get myself back to London.

Some people might have admitted to themselves that there was something seriously wrong with them, and sought help; unaccustomed as I was to relying on others, however, I automatically framed the situation as a major inconvenience certainly, but not one beyond management. With practice, I found that I could stumble along clutching the wall, and was able to shower and dress. By that time, I had learnt to compensate for the continual veering to the left enough to get to breakfast. Despite something in my head not feeling quite right, I found that sitting and slowly eating breakfast were possible. Afterwards, then a smoker and feeling that it might steady me, I lit a cigarette, only to find that I could not direct the ash from my left hand into an ashtray. Instead, seemingly with a life of their own, my fingers were flicking ash all over the table cloth.

Finally, helped by a slight easing of the tendency to lean to port, I learnt to manage my movements well enough to cancel my appointments and snail-pace the drive back to London, where I called in to see my GP. To my dismay, he was very interested in my condition, showed me that my left leg was numb from the knee down by sticking pins in it until the blood ran and finally, called a colleague in to share the excitement. Shortly afterwards, I found

DOI: 10.4324/9781003392088-1

myself at the famous London centre for neurological diseases, the National Hospital, Queen's Square, undergoing a series of tests. I could tell by the sweetness of the nurses' solicitude that I was thought to be in very serious trouble indeed, and this was soon confirmed by the specialist. Pointing out that I was dragging my left foot, he told me that I might well have a very grave illness. A student of psychoanalysis, I queried this – might it not just be an attack of hysterical ataxia? – only to have the doctor tell me that the team thought that I probably had multiple sclerosis, and that my exciting plans to study psychiatric social work in London would have to be put on hold for some time, perhaps for good.

I knew what multiple sclerosis was like from supporting a friend who had contracted it, and the diagnosis filled me with fear and repugnance. I had been sentenced to what, in the 1960s, was a cruel progressive illness, leading inexorably to an early and dreadful end. Above all, I couldn't tell anyone else how terrified I felt about the prospect of the pain and the loss of bodily control that I knew would follow, with death as the only means of escape. As it happened, however, no one asked me how I felt about it.

I also knew that people with multiple sclerosis sometimes lived quite long lives, but how they did it was beyond my imagination. To me, looking on, their lives seemed to be conducted a hair's breadth away from the unendurable. Having hitherto enjoyed excellent health, I did not know then that having a serious disease can still be a way of living, that along with the suffering of the illness and its treatment, there are regular regimens to be undertaken, decisions to be made and activities to be enjoyed. Perhaps felt even more acutely than by the well, the chronically-ill also experience hopes and disappointments and of course, bad times, but there are good times too – time spent with family and friends, or involved in creative projects. Fortunately, the time for me to discover this had not yet come; within weeks, my symptoms had subsided, and finally, disappeared. Twenty years later, a neurosurgeon diagnosed the event retrospectively as the effects of an Oliver Sacks-type, atypical migraine.

In the midst of my relief at having been reprieved, however, a question had formed in my mind which I knew would not leave me until I knew the answer.

How can we move forward from a profound conviction that we must survive at any cost, to accepting that we will die? Is this possible, or do we just resign ourselves to the inevitable?

During the next two decades, I completed a training as a psychotherapist, but even in a world focused on understanding human anguish, my question remained unanswered. Work with the dying was seldom part of a psychotherapist's normal clinical activity; if it was being done at all, this work must largely be taking place somewhere else. In fact, even in ordinary everyday conversation, no one talked about personal death; everyone seemed to know intuitively that it would be a conversation-stopper. Accordingly, when in 1982, a colleague on the board of a respected London hospice offered me the opportunity to volunteer as a psychotherapist there, I accepted without hesitation. Surely, I reflected, for people working with the dying, talking with their patients about how they felt about it would be vital to their care; but it was not so. Perhaps because dying was such an overwhelmingly constant presence, it was not talked about except as a clinical event, in staff meetings. Instead, it was managed by a combination of heavy sedation and pain relief, evangelical services and prayers. I wondered whether, being set apart like that, and all waiting to die, the patients felt isolated or lonely. Did they rebel against dying, or were they just resigned to it? Did they long for someone to keep them company, or to hold their hands until they had taken their last breath? But it was as if a fragile film was holding the routines of the life of the hospice in place, and keeping it intact depended on our being silent about why we were there.

Two further decades passed, and having retired in 2001 from my work as a psychotherapist, I felt a compelling need to discover what my final contribution to this life was to be before it was finally over. I had no idea where to start, but I felt drawn to philosophical inquiry as the royal road to identifying the domain I needed to explore. Since the philosopher's instrument of introspective reflection as the way to understanding the thinking of others was familiar to me from my days as a psychotherapist, I felt at home exploring the minds of Plato and Lucretius, Descartes and Hume, Kant and Thomas Nagel, amongst many others. In 2009, to conclude my studies, I completed an MA by research thesis, in which I defended the radical epistemological sceptic's position that we have no justification for believing that we possess true knowledge about the world we live in. Perhaps fortunately, epistemological scepticism was an unfashionable area of study in philosophical circles then; I eventually discovered that the PhD thesis I planned to write about its roots and continuing ubiquity was not going to be viable.

Into the resultant vacuum, as if it had written itself, a plan for a PhD research thesis proposal to investigate our attitudes to death unfolded in my mind, and I recognised that this was where I wanted to make a final contribution to our understanding of ourselves. However, having assumed that the subject of facing personal death would find a natural home in philosophical circles, I was disappointed to find that death and dying were thought to occupy a highly specialised domain, into which, in 2014, only a very few academic philosophers had ventured. Although there was some interest in areas like ethical issues related to the care of the dying, no philosopher I came across felt able to supervise a study of the experience of personal death as an existential challenge to humanity. Now, I must add here that recently, philosophers have begun to invest significantly in this area of academic investigation, but in those days, the quest to understand what it is like to die would have been much more at home in the domains of sociology or psychology, rather than in philosophy. On the other hand, my inability to find the right place for my PhD proposal did lead me to ask myself some very important and probing questions, questions that all researchers perhaps need to explore before committing themselves to an apparently out-of-left-field project: was my interest in death and dying self-indulgent – perhaps due to some kind of hang-up peculiar to me? Was it time to let it go?

Although I did not know it, what I did need to let go just then was, in fact, the tight control I had been exerting over every phase of my investigation so far; surely, every enterprise needs at some time to make room for the serendipitous, to be open to a possible lucky break. For me, the game-changer came in the very space created by my decision to give up my quest, when a friend suggested that I approach the psychology and counselling branch of Monash University's Education Faculty, to see if they might have a place for my death project on their PhD program. Despite its being at least two standard deviations from the department's norm, in early 2014, Monash University's Education Faculty accepted my project. Even so, as far as I know, there was only one experienced staff member who, although she herself had no background in death studies, was willing to supervise my exploration of it. Catching her in a rare moment of having a vacancy was my second stroke of luck but then, it began to look as though my good fortune had run out.

I could not find a way into death's domain. I did understand that by its nature, research often involves entering previously unknown territory, but as soon as I began to think about who my informants would be, I could see why I seemed to be the first person to study what the dying themselves have to say about the experience of dying. Actually, I had realised those many years ago in the London hospice that the world of the dying is a uniquely private zone; inquisitive outsiders have no place there. As I reflected further on this, I began to feel concerned about my motives for wanting to break into this enclosed domain. Discomfiting questions to which I had no answers then began to badger me; how might my interest in the dying look to them? Was I being voyeuristic, trying to deal vicariously with my own anxieties about dying through investigating the experiences of others? Did I feel like an intruder because I *was* an intruder? Was I a tourist in the kingdom of death, a mere sightseer, blundering about where I did not belong? Again, a question to which I knew I had to find an answer, began to haunt me.

How can I justify entering this sensitive and private zone of which I have no personal experience?

My third stroke of luck arrived at that point, heavily disguised as a tragic blow. Out of the blue, following a bout of pneumonia, and a routine chest X-ray and subsequent CT scan, in early January, 2014, I was diagnosed with metastatic lung cancer, for which there was no worthwhile treatment and which, within months, would lead to a cruel death. I underwent many tests and some harrowing weeks before it was finally discovered that I had again been misdiagnosed. While under sentence of death, however, I had experiences that I believe to have been essential to my acquiring an informed understanding of the travails endured by the participants I later recruited for my study of facing death and equally, to my maintaining a sense of which feeling states belonged to them, and which belonged to me. To record my experience, I kept a journal throughout that time, from which I could potentially draw 'snippets' to enhance or contrast with my participants' material; some of these appear in this book.

Early on in my encounter with death, I had some experiences of altered consciousness in which on a few occasions, I was spoken to by an internal voice which was unfamiliar, but which I understood must belong to me. A significant aspect of the experience of my research participants also, the experience of facing death seems to dissolve some of the forces which normally keep our unconscious processes out of awareness. In my case, the messages came only once, and were brief, authoritative and steadying. For example, on one occasion, when I was struggling to incorporate the diagnosis without panicking, my thoughts suddenly stopped racing and in the pause, a calm and authoritative voice in my head said, "Everything will be fine". I understood that the voice was not saying that I was cancer-free; that was something that I did not know, at any level. Rather, it was telling me that whatever happened, I would find a way to meet it, that my sense of self would not be wiped out. As my study participants also experienced many times, an insightful part of me that I felt I could trust had surfaced. Although 'she' could not know any more than I did about my future, 'she' knew my most basic fear about how the illness might affect me; the reassurance I had received that day never left me. An atheist regarding conventional religious belief, I would not explain these experiences in supernatural terms but equally, I have no wish to repudiate them; I believe that they must come from deep strata in one's own psyche. On the other side of the coin, however, I also endured something of the anguish my participants went through, when I felt the chill of death descend upon me as I lay awake at night and wanted to howl with fear and grief. I also discovered what it was like to feel cosmically alone, no longer a part of everyday mankind, lost in the state that no one wants to talk about.

Eventually, these rehearsals for dying were replaced by an encounter with the real thing. I had known for decades that ischaemic heart disease runs in my family on my father's side and accordingly, when I reached forty, I sought a cardiologist's advice about how best to manage my relatively moderate form of genetically elevated cholesterol. At that time, my cardiologist had told me that the way I would probably die would be not so much from grossly narrowed arteries, as from a piece of arterial plaque breaking off an artery wall and blocking one of my main arteries. Thereafter, I had this prognosis in the back of my mind but in the meantime, I put it aside; I was well, I had no symptoms of heart failure and my blood pressure was enviable for my age. Nonetheless, in mid-2019, I woke up at 4 AM one morning, and without warning – I only subsequently realised that an intermittent pain in my right cheek bone during the previous week had been angina of the jaw – I knew that a catastrophe was taking place in my chest. None of the conventional symptoms of chest pain or breathlessness were present, but the oft-cited 'feeling of doom' was, and it was overwhelming. I called an ambulance, and was taken to hospital.

One of the first things medical staff do is to take a blood test to measure your troponin, the enzyme in the blood which usually becomes elevated when someone is having a heart attack. As my troponin was only mildly elevated, and an X-ray did not reveal damage to my heart, the staff were not sure that there was very much going on. However, blood thinners provided me with so much relief that they decided that they had better keep me in for observation, and sent me to the appropriate ward. Before long, I realised that I was again going downhill quite fast, but the staff could not see it; this was Tuesday evening, and I was told that I would not be having an angiogram until Thursday. It seemed that, although my troponin was more elevated, it was not alarmingly so, and I had only slight and intermittent angina. Nonetheless, I had to tell the nurse that I could feel that I was dying. "Don't say that!", she replied, and then, reassuringly, "Don't worry, you're not dying"; with that, she went off duty.

It is a fact that you can feel the life draining out of you. After a while, I felt no will to further action or agitated concern about what was going to happen. There was only the present, how things were now. As time went on, I began to feel a kind of presence within me, as if some other entity was gradually moving in and spreading out throughout my being; I think of it now as the Great Other. It was certainly disconcerting, but I felt no urge to resist or fight it, though I would have liked someone to have been there to keep me company. But the ward was quiet; it must have been way past midnight, and no one was likely to appear. I felt my fingers brush against the night nurse's buzzer; now on my way out of the world of the living, I had no wish to ring for her, but when I picked the buzzer up and held it, I found it comforting, a kind of instinctive connection with the still living world. Thus anchored, and despite having no idea if I would ever wake up again, I let myself slip away into sleep.

When the night nurse came in at 6 AM and saw how I was, she immediately called the doctor on duty, who ordered a blood test; my troponin level had shot up to dangerous levels. My angiogram was transferred from the following day to first thing that afternoon; when it was carried out, I was found to have an almost complete blockage caused by a piece of plaque having lodged in my left anterior descending artery – the LAD artery, the one known as 'the widowmaker'. The surgeon removed the clot and inserted a stent in the artery. I could feel myself beginning to come back to life.

The dying are not interested in food but the next morning, I ate a meal for the first time in three days. Over the subsequent three years, the stent has settled in well, and though there was some scarring, my heart function has recovered more than the cardiologist had expected. As far as I know, I do not suffer from post-traumatic stress disorder – I do not listen anxiously to my heartbeat or constantly take my blood pressure, for example – and I have completed my PhD degree, and have rewritten my thesis as a book. A little denial in the service of a return to living is a wonderful thing! – but only a little. Too much could be dangerous.

Looking back on my experience of dying from the vantage point of having survived, I have realised that being afraid of death, or filled with sorrow about the final parting with everything that matters, are feelings that belong to being still in the midst of life. By contrast, when I was dying, and knew it, I had no such feelings; embarked on the final journey, I seemed to be spared the anguish of fear and regret about parting with life. Being present during the process of one's dying is completely absorbing; everything else gradually ceases to exist. I believe that the veteran German Jewish sociologist Nobert Elias had it right – dying itself is not necessarily terrible; it is awe-inspiring, profoundly final and nowadays, is often done alone, but it is our natural end: "one passes into dreaming and the world vanishes, if all goes well" (Elias, N. 1985. Loneliness of the dying, p. 66).

In retrospect, I realise that somewhere, sometime, before my confrontation with it, I must have come to accept my own death. I have no memory of doing so, and therefore, no specific awareness of how it came about. I am indebted to my memoirists for showing us the way.

Part II. Humanity cannot face the thought of death

It is time now to move on to the bigger picture, to how other people in advanced societies like our own regard personal death. According to some sociologists, there is a widespread fear of thinking about death amongst us, and becoming more informed about what dying is like is considered the last thing most people would want to do. Rather, focused on survival and ongoing life, mankind is said to turn a blind eye to death and dying, and never more so than when the death concerned is our own. In prospect, death may seem menacing – liable to creep up on us insidiously, and despite our best efforts to resist, to take us away from all that we value and care about. Accordingly, it is usually thought best to avoid it for as long as possible, even though in our depths, we know that inevitably, death is our destiny. On the other hand, since there is no reporting back from the world of the dead, death also holds a certain mystery, even a fascination for us. We might be tempted to watch a sneak preview on reality television about voluntary euthanasia in organisations like Dignitas; occasionally, it is possible even to watch someone die. And yet, while this does prove that death is real and can even be desired, it does not explain how the less willing can come to accept it. Indeed, now that it is quite possible for us to go through life and never come across a death or a corpse, accepting death is becoming increasingly difficult for us even to imagine.

From time immemorial, personal death has posed a challenge to us. Throughout recorded history and in all cultures, the need to survive has been widely considered the instinct most fundamental to all human beings. When we start life as infants, our biological imperative is to thrive within a relationship of attachment; it is not until we are about three years old that we first become conscious of the nature and universality of human death (Norris-Shortle, Young & Williams, 1993). With that discovery, our awareness of the fact that we all die can never be completely lost from our mental life. Rather, the knowledge that our lives must end disappears from consciousness, and typically, becomes alarming or repugnant to it; thereafter, being diagnosed with a terminal illness is arguably the most confronting and enigmatic circumstance that we ever have to face.

In our society, however, death is also a subject that, outside medical circles and health policy, is amongst those topics least talked about; a survey done by Palliative Care Australia a few years ago found that seventy percent of the population believed that we do not talk about death and dying enough (Palliative Care Australia, 2013, p. 1). Including people who are actually facing death, many of us may want to start the conversation, but the rules for doing so, or protocols for finding out if death is a topic our companions would accept, have never been established. Accordingly, without first gaining permission to raise it, stepping into the middle of a social interchange with a question about what dying is like may feel too dangerous to contemplate. And yet, greater freedom to communicate with one another about our death and dying might – amongst other benefits – offer those facing death more opportunities for mutual support, and a better chance of securing excellence in end of life care. At present, perhaps partly because an individual's impending death must first be acknowledged if they are to go to a hospice, only one in four dying Australians are accessing specialist palliative care (Campbell, C., 2018, p. 1).

Without question, then, we need the silence surrounding death and dying in public discourse to be broken. If we are to achieve this, however, we first need information about how to contemplate our mortality – perhaps, stories about people facing death with whom we can identify. As a matter of interest, according to a recent report, educating school children about death is already being considered: "The Australian Medical Association has called for death classes to be implemented in schools to help students deal with the loss of loved ones and their own mortality" (Parenting – School Life, 2018, para. 1). Now, in advocating public education about death and dying, I am not suggesting that the best way to inform people would be to provide them with a dissertation on death as such, or on being dead. Rather, the objective would be to open up the conversation about the human experience of facing death, and how this most significant moment in our lives can be further understood, enriched and humanised.

Almost immediately I had conceived it, my intention of producing a book for myself, as well as for the public to gain some understanding of what dying is like, faced an apparently insuperable challenge. How could I find people to interview who would be willing to tell me, in their own words, about their experience of dying? To carry out such a study would be impractical, and very likely, unethical. As an alternative, I could interview fit and well volunteers about how they felt about the *prospect* of death as the eventual end to their lives; this could be interesting and worthwhile, but it fell short of what I had in mind. As my thoughts wandered, I found myself pausing over recollections of some remarkable memoirs that I had read, journals written by people who were actually facing death in the comparatively near future. All of these memoirists were accomplished writers, and the way they described their experiences of grappling with the diagnosis, the illness and its treatment, and finally, the approach of death, was accessible and powerful. Accordingly, I decided that it would be just as productive to focus on these memoirs as research data for my book, as it would be to interview living people, whether well or terminally-ill.

There were two main advantages to using these memoirs as data sources. Firstly, the fact that all of the authors were now deceased simplified the ethical issues which usually characterise this kind of research. Although it would be necessary to seek permission to use quotations from the memoirs through consultation with their authors' copyright holders, they were already published, and generally available. By contrast, even if it were possible to collect, any research material obtained from interviews with the dying would be sensitive not only after they had died, but even more so while they were still alive; a wide range of ethical issues would have to be considered. Indeed, permission to carry out the research might turn out to be impossible to obtain. And there was another consideration; using memoirs for my research data would allow a detailed, longitudinal study to be done about the experience of preparing for death, from the time of the original diagnosis, right through to the end of life. Data such as this may not have been possible to retrieve from face-to-face interviews.

Accordingly, having reviewed my options, I decided make use of memoirs by the dying to provide the data I needed to research the 'burning questions' on which my proposed book would be based. Given that the book would not be an investigation of attitudes to personal death and dying across a whole population but rather, an exploratory inquiry, examining in depth the subjective experience of a small group of people with terminal illnesses, the memoirs were exactly what was wanted. As everything seemed to be coming together at last, I could give the book a provisional title: *End of life experience: Facing death*, and by now fully unpacked, the questions it was intended to address were:

1 ***What is it like to face death?***
2 ***If our most basic instinct is to survive, how can we become ready to relinquish life and accept death?***

Reflecting on the second question, I realised that there was a perplexing conundrum implied by Question 2, which would need to be resolved:

There is a paradox at the heart of human existence which contains two fundamental but apparently incompatible truths:

i) Our most basic instinct is to survive, and to avert death at all costs
ii) We know throughout life that we must die

Upon further analysis, Question 2 was found to contain four implied sub-questions, which the book would need to address:

a) Do we ever accept that we must die? Or do we simply succumb to it when death finally overtakes us?
b) Can the paradox of existence be resolved? Or do we finally come to an understanding of our mortality which allows the paradox to disperse?

Finding a way to resolve the paradox is not just an academic exercise. Its origin lies in our very make-up, in the fact that human beings possess reflexive consciousness; since we are capable of mentally observing our own thoughts as if from a position slightly outside them, we can evaluate what any particular proposition means to us in the context of our other concerns. Accordingly, when the thought that we will die comes to mind, it will routinely evoke the paradox which underlies it, and arguably, the less first-hand experience we have with how death can be met with acceptance, the more likely we will be to come down on the side of seeking to prolong life at all costs. Indeed, it is not unusual nowadays to hear or read reports purporting to be scientifically-based declaring that reasonably soon, we will not have to die at all. For example, as far back as 1999, science and popular fiction writer, Damien Broderick, received high praise from respected book reviewers and some academics for his book *The last mortal generation*, which opened with the claim that: "Sometime in the twenty-first century, ordinary humans like you and me – or our children and grandchildren – will be offered new medical treatments that will lead, eventually, to physical immortality" (Broderick, 1999, p. 1).

Arguably, people in comparatively affluent and scientifically sophisticated societies are vulnerable to uncritical acceptance of this kind of claim. However, even if we are aware of the danger of locking ourselves into such an impossible and unaffordable aspiration, we are not necessarily ready to embrace the alternative of working towards a timely death. If that is not possible and therefore, the paradox cannot be resolved, the whole dilemma is liable to be suppressed from our collective consciousness. If that were to be the case, any programs which rely for success on a widespread grasp of the reality of our mortality, and a sense of shared responsibility for it – for example, Advance Care Planning – are likely to continue to be generally avoided. Unfortunately, there is no obvious answer to this conundrum, and like all tough and controversial issues, if not freely aired, it is liable, eventually, to disappear unresolved from public debate. But one thing is certain; if we choose to believe that we will never have to die, it may in time become grotesque, even offensive, for anyone to mention the natural process of dying in ordinary conversation, and if that became the case, our commitment to seeking its best practice management would also be difficult to sustain.

Let us suppose that when we think about it, we do not want to find ourselves in such a hazardous position. To whom might we turn to keep the conversation about death and dying observant of tradition and yet, contemporary? At first glance, it may seem to make sense to assign this weighty task to the medical profession; as they have the expertise in illness and terminal conditions, perhaps we should give them permission to undertake some public education, as well as to raise the subject with patients. But is this to expect more of doctors than they are at present qualified to do? It cannot just be assumed that their training in how to keep people alive also gives them the background in, and confidence to engage people in conversations about how they are likely to die. Therefore, it is encouraging to note that within the last few years, some determined moves towards addressing this issue are taking place at least in some Intensive Care Unit wards. For example, Victorian ICU specialist, Dr Charlie Corke, recognises that the dying value honest conversation with their physician – even, or perhaps especially, at the last; he has written a book about his work entitled *Letting go,* and with his colleague, Ken Hillman, he has also been broadcasting about it (Corke, 2018).

In the final analysis, however, keeping the conversation about death and dying from slipping away from us is going to be largely up to us. It is in the service of our shouldering this responsibility that I am writing this book. It is not for all communities; it is intended primarily for societies like my own, societies I have referred to in this chapter as 'advanced'. My use of the word 'advanced' acknowledges that the findings in my study and the views and theories I refer to apply only to individuals in societies like my own Australian community – societies such as Canada, the UK, Europe, North America and New Zealand. While far from being homogeneous cultures, these societies have many practices in common, including their management of death and dying. The practices of other very different communities – Indian, Middle Eastern or Chinese cultures, for example – are very different both from mine and from each other, and a few token paragraphs about the practices of some of them would not do them justice; therefore, I have not included any. I have no doubt that a discussion of the approach to death and dying in each of these cultures would require a volume of its own.

The five memoirists who have provided us with such invaluable data about their experience of dying all died of natural causes, and were in their sixties and seventies; this is not a book about people who die young, though such a study is also needed. By its nature, it is as well a book about educated, middle-class people; it does not draw on the experience of the working class – a study that is also needed. A small exploratory study which is not generalisable, this book is intended to open up a conversation which in time, will extend and enrich the horizons of our thinking about death and dying.

Finally, I owe the memoirists my heartfelt thanks for their unique and generous contribution to our understanding. To be more completely introduced in Chapter 4, with their stories about dying told in the following chapters, they are:

English writer, Jenny Diski, who died in 2016 aged 68. Her 2016 memoir is *In gratitude.*

English political strategist for New Labour, Lord Philip Gould, Baron Brookwood, who died in 2011, aged 61. His 2012 memoir is *When I die: Lessons from the Death Zone.*

English/American public intellectual and writer, Christopher Hitchens, who died in 2011, aged 62. His 2012 memoir is *Mortality.*

English clergyman, The Very Reverend Michael Mayne, Dean Emeritus of Westminster, who died in 2006, aged 77. His 2006 memoir is *The Enduring Melody.*

Australian writer, Cory Taylor, who died in 2016, aged 61. Her 2016 memoir is *Dying: A memoir.*

References

Broderick, D. (1999). *The last mortal generation.* Australia: New Holland Press.

Campbell, C. (2018). SA failed to uphold pledge to improve palliative care report. *ABC Radio National AM Program Report.* Retrieved from https://www.abc.net.au/radio/programs/am/sa-failed-to-uphold-pledge-to-improve-pallitative-care-report/10645236

Corke, C. (2018). *Letting go: How to plan for a good death.* London and Brunswick, Melbourne: Scribe Books.

Diski, J. (2016). *In gratitude.* London and New York: Bloomsbury Publishing.

Elias, N. (1985). *The loneliness of the dying.* E. Jephcott (Trans.). Oxford: Basil Blackwell Ltd.

Gould, P. (2013). *When I die: Lessons from the death zone.* London: Abacus, Little, Brown Book Group.

Hitchens, C. E. (2012). *Mortality.* New York, Boston, MA: Twelve Books.

Mayne, M. C. O. (2006). *The enduring melody.* London: Darton, Longman and Todd.

Norris-Shortle, C., Young, P. A., & Williams, M. A. (1993). Understanding death and grief for children three and younger. *Social Work 38* (6), 736–742. https://academic.oup.com/sw

Palliative Care Australia (2013). *Election platform.* Retrieved 15/12/13 from http://www.palliativecare.org.au/Portals/46/Election%202007/Election/202013/PCA%20 Election20Statements.pdf

Parenting – School Life. (2018, May, 25). Death classes: Queensland schools encouraged to implement lessons about mortality. *News.com.au,* 25/05/18. Retrieved from https://www.news.com.au/lifestyle/parenting/schools-life/death-class-qld-schools-encouraged-implement-lessons-about-mortality/news-story/2406b9aae78ebc483d10be655f093a2f

Taylor, C. (2016). *Dying: A memoir.* Melbourne: Text Publishing.

2 Death as enigma

Introduction: When does dying become death?

Ongoing debates exist about non-heart-beat protocols for determining the 'irreversible' moment of death, and this is one reason for its being difficult even for experienced doctors to predict. For some, the complex reality that is death is best defined as "the loss of the organism as a whole" – usually referred to as "passed" or "passed away" – while for others, death is more precisely defined as "loss of consciousness or personhood", less widely known as "de-animation" (Shewmon, 2010, p. 1). For the purposes of this investigation, however, a broadly-based existential description of death over time is more appropriate than either of these definitions: "Death is defined as the permanent cessation of purposeful adaptive interaction with the environment ... followed by disintegration of our organs and cells" (Bartalos, 2008, p. 194).

Australian sociologist Alan Kellehear (2014) sees dying as taking place over an extended period, perhaps even years, rather than during the last few minutes of someone's life. When a condition is terminal but death is not yet imminent, the awareness that they are dying may not always be in the forefront of a person's mind. Accordingly, with time in hand, they have the chance to reflect on the meaning of their lives and perhaps, to complete some long-cherished project, before making their final farewells. The memoir-writing participants in this study exemplify this kind of dying.

The chapter is divided into three parts, as follows:

Part I. We cannot conceive of our own death
Part II. The taboo on talking about personal death
Part III. Turning a blind eye to death: The sequestration of the dying

Part I. We cannot conceive of our own death

As long ago as the early seventeenth century, La Rochefoucauld observed: "Neither the sun nor death can be looked at steadily". In fact, there is an insurmountable barrier to our being able to imagine ourselves dead; in the very act of trying to do so, we cannot help demonstrating that since we are imagining something, we are still alive. As noted by Polish sociologist, Zygmunt

DOI: 10.4324/9781003392088-2

Baumann: "Death cannot be perceived; still less visualised or 'represented' … death is the cessation of the very 'acting subject' and with it, the end of all perception"; the perceiving subject "cannot 'blot itself out' of the perception and still wish the perception to be" (Bauman, 1992, pp. 1–2).

But La Rochefoucauld thinks that there is another, more willed, dimension to our blind spot about death; he is suggesting that the fear of being overwhelmed by it makes us avoid even trying to picture ourselves facing imminent death. Often quoted still, La Rochefoucauld's aphorism remains unchallenged. However, a good deal has been written about the whys and wherefores of our fear of personal death, and our aversion to thinking about it; these barriers to our thinking about death fall into two broad categories, the cognitive-perceptual, and the emotional.

Cognitive-perceptual difficulties in conceptualising one's own death

Zygmunt Bauman has devoted a book to trying to understand the nature of human death and how comprehensively our foreknowledge of it affects us, both individually, and within our social institutions. He argues that in modernity, death has become an unmanageable void with which we can cohabit only by forgetting about it (Bauman, 1992). Similarly, Clive Seale describes us as living with our prospective mortality in a state of persistent unawareness (Seale, 1998, p. 177). For Bauman and Seale, the sequestration of the dying and the dead described later in the chapter, can be understood as representing the way we dissociate from knowing about personal death in order to maintain the illusion of a never-ending future. On this view, the awareness that eventually, we will have to face death, is packed away in a compartment of our minds which we hope will never have to be opened. Sooner or later, though, we will be confronted with death – perhaps first, through seeing a loved one die – and be forced to acknowledge that dying is an inescapable reality that someday, we will have to reckon with. We will also discover that seeing others die tells us very little about how we will meet the challenge of dying ourselves.

As Bauman observes: "Death is the absolute Other of being, an unimaginable other, hovering beyond the reach of communication … Death is not like other others, which the eye is free to fill with meaning and to constitute – and subordinate" (Bauman, 1992, p. 2). Given that it has no existential aftermath, our personal death is the only experience we will ever have which, once it is over, we cannot then characterise, and discuss with similarly-experienced others. As science journalist Robin Henig points out: "There is only one chance [to die] … and there is no reporting back from the field" (Henig, 2005, p. 13). Accordingly, since personal death cannot be symbolised within a shared language, it eludes our control. Impossible to label, classify, and file away, it cannot be mastered, and thus, kept under our collective thumb.

Emotional difficulties in conceptualising one's own death

In *The loneliness of the dying*, Norbert Elias observes that, while the pacification of modern societies has removed the violence and brutishness from everyday life, it has also done away with our everyday experience of contact with the dying. We are left with little shared sense of death's meaning for us, no meta-narrative to identify it communally, and as a consequence, few agreed rituals with which to contain its impact upon us. Our lack of experience of death as a reality leaves us vulnerable to the fears and fantasies of our particular culture – perhaps that death will find us helpless and terrified, left to die alone in uncontrollable pain and suffering or perhaps, prey to menacing hallucinations of being taken by some kind of dreaded presence like the Grim Reaper. Finally, there is the fear of losing everything we treasure about being alive. A number of studies report that while we are still well, amongst the items we fear losing when we die – loved ones, feeling connected to our sentient groups, and the sheer joy of living – the fear of losing our everyday sense of self in relationships with others ranks high (Elias, 1985; Feifel, 1959; Becker, 1973; Di Masi, 2004). In this connection, it is interesting to recall that my own experience when actually dying, was not like that; fear and regret about parting with the precious things in life did not arise. As I reported in Chapter 1: "Being present during the process of one's dying is completely absorbing; everything else gradually ceases to exist". I had reflected then that perhaps fear and regret about dying are felt more by those still in the midst of life.

There is another kind of fear of death, a fear related to its unique strangeness, to its being something utterly alien to our lived experience. Canadian philosopher Kathy Behrendt claims that because it represents non-existence, or nothingness, death arouses a special kind of fear in us. She holds that, although it is of "an anomaly, untethered to an image", the fear of non-existence is a true fear, albeit of an "abstract propositional conception" (Behrendt, 2010, p. 677). Just as the thought of some unimaginable alternative reality taking over our planet frightens us, so too does the idea of non-existence. Since neither can be imagined nor rendered intelligible in the perceptual-centred, cognitivist framework of our everyday world, we find ourselves lost for words, overtaken by the uncanny. Try as we might to tell ourselves that of course, we all know perfectly well that we must die, according to Behrendt, this kind of objectively-minded self is not in a position of safety when contemplating death. In fact, she agrees with philosopher Thomas Nagel's view that: "'[W]e cannot rise above death by occupying a vantage point that death will destroy'" (Behrendt, 2010, p. 681).

In all, given our inability to imagine, or to find our own death symbolisable, it is ultimately rendered literally "unthinkable". For most people, even if it turns out to be illusory, being able to put into words a feeling or an intuition about something that has been bothering us, gives us a sense of mastery. Accordingly, our inability to identify what death *is* – as opposed to what it *does* – only makes it seem the more threatening; it is so very final and yet, it is forever beyond our control. No matter how alert and fit we are, in the ordinary way, we cannot choose when it will happen, or exert any influence over whether it will be kind or terrible.

Unwilling to accept this prevailing view of our mortality, however, Italian psychoanalyst Franco Di Masi asks whether it is possible to make death "thinkable".

Di Masi: Making death "thinkable"

Observing that for many of us, death is unthinkable and yet, it is real, Di Masi's take on death as an "absent presence … [and an] unsymbolisable nothingness" (Di Masi, 2004, p. 111), resonates with both Behrendt's and Bauman's positions. He quotes studies in neuroscience which corroborate his clinical findings that, by stimulating mechanisms that inhibit explicit memory processes, very frightening memories cause dissociation, a blockage of the capacity to recall those memories. In this way, traumatic experiences are separated from the rest of the psyche, "allowing the victim to function as if the trauma had never happened" (Di Masi, 2004, p. 114). According to Di Masi, this process also allows us to remain unaware of the paradox of our existence – that at one and the same time, we can know that we are transient and yet, maintain the illusion of our capacity for infinite development. But Di Masi is more optimistic than Bauman about our capacity for undoing damaging repressions and accepting that our lives are finite. He suggests that education is necessary to counter the infantile belief that we are exempt from death. Beginning with children, its objective would be to introduce us to the psychic work that we need to do to be ready to acknowledge the prospect of death, while at the same time, committing ourselves to living life to the full. In conclusion, Di Masi argues that we should be encouraged to recognise that, even though death is inscribed in our internal world as a state of disintegration of our personal identity, nonetheless – going against our usual estimation of our capacities – "we have the emotional resources necessary … to limit and contain the feelings of loneliness and the pain of death" (Di Masi, 2004, p. 26). Indeed, if we think about it, many of us know personally people who have looked death in the eye, but have neither determined to put it out of their minds, nor been overwhelmed by it.

To sum up: repression need not be our only way of coping with death or with the prospect of dying which, for some people, is even more frightening than death.

Part II. The taboo on talking about personal death

A significant body of opinion holds that, due to our inability to conceptualise our own death, we cannot communicate with one another about it. For these observers, if silence does surround the subject of our own death, our inability to express and hence, to share what our death means to us would be the reason for it. On this view, our silence about death is essentially the result of a conceptual hiatus; we simply do not have the tools to talk about it.

By contrast, some social commentators claim that the absence of reference to personal death in everyday conversation does not originate in a conceptual problem; they argue that there is a taboo in place against talking about death that is so powerful that we are afraid to raise the subject. Others again would argue that this view is too extreme; according to them, our steering clear of mentioning death in ordinary social interchanges is just a matter of normal conversational etiquette. According to them, one simply needs to have the good manners to choose an appropriate moment to raise possibly awkward subjects like personal death, just as one would exercise caution about bringing up intimate details of one's marital problems.

Does this view about the absence of death from everyday conversation really account for it? Or does our silence about death come from depths far more primitive and fearful than the dictates of social correctness? If so, talking about death would not be discouraged merely because it would be embarrassing; it would indicate the presence of a taboo so powerful that referring to it in ordinary conversation has become absolutely forbidden.

What, then, is the truth of the matter?

Tony Walter: Talking about death is difficult, but it is not taboo

English sociologist Tony Walter distinguishes a weak sense of 'taboo' from its stronger counterpart as follows:

> In everyday usage, the word 'taboo' refers to something prohibited, forbidden by custom rather than by law. It may be something that is too terrible to think of, its reality denied. Or, more weakly, it simply may not be mentioned in conversation.
>
> (Walter, 1991, p. 295)

He argues that referring to death and dying in everyday conversation is comparable to referring to one's sex life, or addiction to drugs; it is merely subject to everyday conversational norms regarding appropriate time and place. On reflection, he decides that there are no taboo aspects of talking about death; it is merely a socially constrained, rather than a forbidden domain (Walter, 1991, p. 307).

There are two main arguments from other specialists which support Walter's claim. The first relates to our society's expectation of reticence and emotional continence in all social contexts. According to American historian, Peter Stearns (1994), death is just one of many subjects which, since the transition away from the emotional expressiveness of Victorian times, are now generally thought to be best not mentioned. Stearns contends that by the late twentieth century, it was generally believed that talking about death should be kept clear of the so-called "negative emotions" like uncontrolled sorrow, anger and fear, and instead, associated with happier themes, like eulogies for the departed which, informally and often humorously, celebrate their lives (Stearns, 1994, pp. 161–162); this trend has continued and indeed, flourished.

Secondly, from a different angle, there are anthropologists who argue that the silence about personal death has never been dictated by conversational etiquette or taboos but rather, is an effect of the conceptual difficulties of talking about death discussed in the previous section. On this view, people may hesitate to talk about personal death either because they lack the right words to do so, or because they anticipate receiving an uncomprehending stare in response. Some scholars would argue further that, due to the loss of religion-based frameworks within which to think about our own death, we have been silenced where once we could communicate freely. Whatever the reason, the result is the same; as we no longer have a shared way to understand and conceptualise the nature of personal death, we cannot talk to each other about it.

And yet, exceptions to this can be found; under certain specific circumstances, people who need to do so, and who have experienced, and are again experiencing immediate threats to their lives, do find a way to talk about it.

A shared language about death can develop in specialised settings

Israeli anthropologist, Tova Gamliel, has found that the spontaneous development of a shared language about personal death can occur in a particular population. Also noting that in general, we lack the concepts or symbolic discourse to relate to our own death, Gamliel studied two hundred and thirty European Jews living in an Israeli aged care facility, in order to find out if they had found a way specific to them, to talk about illness and death. Within this specialised domain, Gamliel (2008) found that, drawing on their shared culture and history, these elderly people had developed a framework which had rendered it both socially acceptable and conceptually possible to talk about death. Given that their impending death was the one subject which provided the residents with some sense of solidarity, they had developed a private language to talk about it; Gamliel called it "the danse macabre" (p. 261). In comparison with the 'objective' discourse of academics on the subject, the talk which developed among her elderly subjects was subjective, value-laden and above all, situated in a particular social world. For example, they referred to their own deaths as "disappearances", and also using Nazi terminology: "There's always a transport" or, "We're up for liquidation". They described each other as "stiffs", and "already circling the drain"; in the mornings, they would open someone's door, and shout: "Good morning – just to see if you're alive!" (Gamliel, 2008, pp. 265–267). A kind of naturalism which aims to diminish the horrific impression of death by emphasising its universality and necessity, it goes against the grain of modern mythology's notion of a 'good death' because it does not seek to blunt death's pernicious outcome; far from hiding the more terrible aspects of dying, this 'danse macabre' highlights them. Residents could use their command of this vernacular to rebel against the rational discourse of authority, standard linguistic usage and especially, against their fate, and enjoy "a chuckle in the face of death" (Gamliel, 2008, p. 272).

As Gamliel observes, all meaning requires an overarching communication protocol which is atemporal and impersonal, but in order to be functional, it must also relate to the life experience of the population it serves. Talk about death at a high level of abstraction in academic research, medical management or government policy, or at a distance in news bulletins, is routine nowadays. By contrast, Gamliel's research shows that, when ordinary people are obliged to talk personally about *my* death and *your* death, they have to adapt everyday language to meet their specific subjective needs to understand, and be understood; the pre-requisite to doing so is shared experience and awareness at depth of what it is like facing death. Limited to small localised groups, such exchanges may only occasionally be possible in the everyday social intercourse of modern society.

Contra Walter: There is a taboo on talking about death

Contra Walter's position, there is still a widely held belief in our society that a taboo does exist on talking about death. There are two main arguments in favour of this view also. The first, advanced by Gamliel, suggests that a possible reason for the silence surrounding death is that it is assumed to be an issue mainly for the elderly; she argues that the silence is a logical extension of a general view of the elderly as best ignored, as "culturally invisible .... [Their] voice ... is seldom heard" (Gamliel, 2008, p. 262). In support of this view, both American social work academic Davis-Berman (2011, p. 365) and Canadian sociologists Clarke, Korotchenko and Bundon report being told that, when the elderly aged care residents whom they interviewed on their attitudes to death and dying had previously sought the opportunity to talk about their approaching death, nobody in their facilities had been willing to listen (Clarke et al., 2012, p. 1411). Arguably, however, this 'silencing' is not necessarily directed at the elderly *per se*. Rather, it is specifically directed at their wish to talk about death; their interest in discussing other topics was accepted. Similarly, a study by American communication analysts Caughlin, Mikucki-Enyart, Middleton, Stone, and Brown of how members of the families of terminal lung cancer patients handled the subject of the illness showed that, although some family members wanted to talk openly about the impending death, they were silenced by others who believed that this would "just upset everyone" and "saddle them with other people's lack of self-control" (Caughlin et al., 2011, Emotional avoidance). Arguably, in both examples, a reality too disturbing to articulate had to be suppressed; that is the function of a taboo.

Conceding that a taboo of sorts might exist on talking about death, Walter observes that if there is a taboo on talking about death, hospital staff dedicated to keeping people alive, rather than society at large, would be responsible for its existence; he quotes Kellehear's (1984) opinion that patients are "too embarrassed" to talk to doctors about dying (Walter, 1991, p. 302). As described in Chapter 1, when, during my stay in hospital, I told the nurse that I believed that I was dying, she exclaimed: "Don't say that!" – and went off duty. Certainly, following a blood test of my troponin level early the next morning, my angiogram had been brought forward as urgent. Nonetheless, when I had told the nurse that I felt that I was dying, there was no conversation, and no checking out of what I had said; I was simply shut down. What Kellehear had said over thirty years earlier about patients believing that medical professionals can be averse to being talked to about their dying may still be the case. If so, it could represent a serious risk to life.

How might such an unfortunate situation have come about? In an article entitled: "Why we don't talk about death and dying", Australian ethicist and legal academic, Malcolm Parker (2011), observes that, although ICU medical staff have recently spearheaded a move for change in the 'keep treating, never give up' tradition of hospital doctors, the practice continues, and crucial end of life conversations still may not be possible. In Parker's opinion: "There's said to be a measure of collusion between society and medicine, orchestrated via the media's unrealistic and unbalanced portrayal of medical progress and success" (p. 4). This practice is highly resistant to change; not long ago, ICU consultant, Charlie Corke, was still finding himself grappling every day with the task of making room in the constant treatment activities, for the vital end of life conversations his dying patients urgently needed to have (Corke, 2018).

The silence must end: Talking about death is essential

Whatever the academic debates about the nature of the silence about death, the media have been in no doubt that it is due to the existence of a taboo. In mid-2019, the following excerpts were among the first of many which appeared on the internet in response to the words, 'taboo on talking about death' being typed into the browser.

> In 2017, the UK Marie Curie hospice organisation declared: "Our reluctance to talk about death risks leaving us vulnerable and underprepared. The uncomfortable truth is this: ... death is something we all have to face, whether our own or others".
>
> (Marie Curie, 2017 blog, 2017, "Help us break the taboo around death?" para 1)

> In 2018, BBC News quoted the Sue Ryder charity for palliative support as follows: "A charity is calling for a 'national conversation' about dying, saying the topic has become 'taboo' and a source of anxiety for many".
>
> (BBC News, Health, 2018, para 1)

> By 2019, some progress on the issue was being made; in the popular health journal, *Psychology Today*, Marc Whitman asked: "Is there a taboo on talking about death? A line of thought in Western culture argues in favour of this idea".
>
> (Whitman, 2019, para. 1)

> After some discussion, however, Whitman suggests tentatively that while there are still many deniers, more people are becoming willing to confront our mortality.

In fact, the taboo or restraint said to exist on talking about death has recently been reported by various agencies as beginning to come under pressure. Investigating the fear of death presumed to lie behind the silence about it, Netherlands clinical psychologist research team De Raedt, Koster and Ryckewaert found that older adults were less inclined to avoid death-related threats brought to their attention than younger adults were. As Gamliel had also discovered, they suggest that with aging, talk of death is less avoided, and that this may indicate greater acceptance of one's own finiteness in old age (De Raedt et al., 2013, p. 41). In the following year, Palliative Care Australia conducted a survey which revealed that 70% of Australians believed that we do not talk about death and dying enough; PCA suggested that government install a dedicated telephone line for people to access if they wanted to talk about it (PCA, 2013, p. 2). A year later, John Troyer, an academic developing a program to harvest organs for transplant purposes, claimed that death and dying are no longer forbidden topics in the same way as for example, necrophilia is:

> Why are so many academics and commentators so committed to saying that death is a socially repressed topic? All that most people need to talk about death-topics is a bit of encouragement.
>
> (Troyer, 2014, p. 2)

But changing an ingrained social custom is never easy, and requires strategies to be put in place. Usually, there is a group or groups who want a particular change, and others who oppose it; this was seen clearly in the recent legislation for same-sex marriage in Australia. Similarly, research by Davis-Berman, Clark et al., Caughlin et al., and the researcher's hospital experience, show that neither conversational etiquette nor lack of language resources were the immediate cause of preventing those who really wanted to talk about death and dying from doing so; in fact, they were being actively silenced or ignored by other people who had the power to do it. Given that those who were reported as being shut down were either in a family setting, or in hospital or residential aged care facilities, this shutting-down of free expression by the more powerful seems to reflect a determination to suppress activities that they think could have emotive and unpredictable effects on the institution's functioning.

But there is a misdirection of attention involved here; although the avoided subject is usually said to be 'death', or 'death and dying' in general, perhaps this large canvas is a screen to hide something far more specific. Arguably, what crucially must not be mentioned is the approaching death of *someone in particular,* of *your* death or *my* death. In Caughlin's study of the families of terminal lung cancer patients, the crux of the matter was spelt out; in order to avoid "just upsetting everyone", silence about the forthcoming death of an *identified terminally-ill family member* was what was required. Of course, one of our greatest anxieties concerns the potential loss of a loved one, but lying just beyond, and because it means the loss of everything we care about, the greatest threat of all is the death of the self.

Defining a strong taboo as applying only to "Something that is too terrible to think of, its reality denied", Walter (1991, p. 295) has claimed that there is not even a weak taboo on talking about personal death; rather, in the same way as talk of sex or drug-taking is regulated, talking about death is governed by rules of conversational etiquette. Arguably, however, in contemporary society, if the conversation does ever move towards areas like the death of particular persons, it will almost certainly be diverted to safer topics. Whether it amounts to a taboo or not, perhaps the restraint on talk of death in general is a tacit back-up provision, intended to prevent us from even approaching the real danger zone, the death of the self.

On the other hand, if our need to talk about death and dying is now becoming greater than our fear of it, the next move most likely lies in public education, and according to some, as shown in the following excerpts, children should be involved from the beginning.

Suggested programs for public education about death: Focus on children and young people

On May 25th, 2018, it was announced on News. com: "The Australian Medical Association has called for death classes to be implemented in schools to help students deal with the loss of loved ones and their own mortality" (News.com.au., 2018, May 25, para. 1). ICU consultant Charlie Corke also believes from long experience of working with the dying and their families, that people should be encouraged to think about death and dying at school (Corke & Hillman, 2018, Radio interview).

On July, 30th, 2018, following a successful Dying Matters week in May, NHS Gateshead Health in the UK initiated a project to break down the taboo on talking about death and dying with children. Links were forged with the local secondary school to encourage children to talk about death, and to support each other when their family members, teachers or school friends were faced with a palliated illness. Speaking about the outcome of the project, the project leader said:

> It was such a privilege to speak to the children and get their views on three important questions as below:
>
> 1 Should children be involved in discussions about death, dying and bereavement?
> 2 What would you say or do for someone who had just lost somebody?
> 3 What would you want somebody to say or do for you if you had just lost somebody?
>
> The replies were overwhelming, and showed that children do want to be involved in these conversations, and need to be.
>
> (https://www.hospiceuk.org/our-campaigns/dying-matters)

Evaluating the debate

In claiming that in modern society, reticence about personal death is in the same category as reticence about our sex lives or drug-taking habits, Walter suggests that talk about personal death is avoided in everyday social contexts because it causes embarrassment (Walter, 1991, p. 295). But would expressing one's concerns about dying be unsuitably revealing in the same way as giving someone a hands-on account of one's most recent sexual encounter? Arguably, rather than embarrassing us, talk of someone's dying or grave illness may make us feel completely out of our depth, because we have no idea what to say. Talking about *my* death, or *your* death seems to be closer to exposing "a reality too terrible to think about" than to precipitating a mere conversational glitch. Ensuring that it does not arise in the first place, social custom now deems talking about death to be in poor taste; accordingly, most people can be relied upon not to introduce it into everyday conversation.

Of course, there are subjects related to death and dying which are regularly talked about – for example, practical matters like wills, finances, costs, celebrants and churches, obituaries, and the procedure for a funeral. These topics are safe; they are practical, and have known limits. By contrast, talking about personal death is hazardous, its boundaries unknown and its depths feared to be a repository for the too-confronting. On the other hand, there are signs that more and more people do not want to remain silenced and intimidated; perhaps beginning to introduce our children into a world in which death and dying are more freely explored will help to open the subject up for future generations.

Part III. Turning a blind eye to death: The sequestration of the dying

In earlier centuries, death from accident or illness was often clearly observable and soon over. In modern society, however, as noted earlier in this chapter, advances in medical science and technology have made dying a more drawn-out and unpredictable process. As American philosopher William Gavin observes:

> The passing of the person is being lost in clinical processes … [and in] a complex of organs and machines. The moment of passing does not happen, and so cannot be prepared for or ritualized.
>
> (Gavin, 1995, p. 29)

Such a death often requires that in their final hours, the dying individual is sequestered away from their loved ones, to permit a final round of life-saving efforts in hospital ICUs. More generally, the level of medicalisation in our society's end of life care makes the sequestration of some chronically-ill and frail elderly people inevitable; for some commentators, no further explanation of sequestration practices is needed. For others, though, such practices are also to be understood firstly, as expressions at the societal level of our need to remain unaware of our mortality, and secondly, as a means of protecting us from witnessing the suffering that may be in store for us because of modern medicine's obligation to keep us alive.

Sequestration defined

Opinions vary on what exactly constitutes the sequestration of death and dying in modern society; a definition offered by British sociologist Glennys Howarth focuses on the withdrawal of death and dying from public space and awareness:

> A number of sociologists have argued that in contemporary Western societies – broadly depicted as 'postmodern' or 'high modern' – death has been *sequestered* (Howarth's emphasis). By this they mean that death has been removed from the public sphere and located instead in the private world of the individual. This [term]... explains the ... apparent absence of death in the public realm and the presence of death in the private lives of individuals.... Sequestration is illustrated in that the majority of people now die in institutions, away from the public gaze.
>
> (Howarth, 2007a, pp. 23–24)

Representing a second approach, British nursing academic Katherine Froggatt provides a more operational view:

> Sequestration is the term for the process of setting apart or separating out. It is used in two ways regarding sickness and death – i) at a societal level, it is used to describe the way in which modern society has set death apart from our ordinary lives, perhaps through the use of organisations, and ii) as the model which explains the separation of defined groups within an institution, as perceived, the dying from the living, or the unbounded bodies from the bounded ones.
>
> (Froggatt, 2001, p. 320)

The first definition demonstrates the common, if perhaps confusing use of 'public' and 'private' in describing the change from traditional ways of managing death and dying within the community, to their present-day management in specialised institutions; the second definition provides an operational description of the two different approaches social theory brings to its analysis.

Death and dying have vanished from everyday life

We have become unfamiliar with death and dying. In the UK, before the Second World War, a sixteen year-old would have seen on average at least six people die, whereas now it is possible to arrive at fifty without ever having seen a corpse (Ballatt & Campling, 2011, p. 116). In Australia, the statistics are likely to be similar. In general, our society's experience of encountering mortality has changed radically since the beginning of the twentieth century ushered in "a diversity of contemporary deathways" (Hockey, 2007, p. 436). Two such changes include the previously-mentioned medicalisation and sequestration of death, as well as the loss of religious meta-narratives about its meaning. A third concerns the way we maintain our acquaintance with the fact that death exists. English sociologist Geoffrey Gorer (1955/1994) has claimed that, inclined as we are to divert our attention away from flesh-and-blood death, we have for decades been provided with ample opportunity to contemplate it as the death of the other, viewed at a safe distance through its depiction in the media. In *The pornography of death*, Gorer argues that what is unacceptable to us about death – its ugliness and its deadly power – now largely appears onscreen, in graphic depictions of murders and sadistic violence in films, or even in the daily television news (Gorer, 1955/1994).

Our dissociation from the reality of death has not been intentional. Rather, it is the ultimate result of the medicalisation of death, a process which has gathered momentum exponentially since transfers of the sick from home to hospital began in the 1930s, and became widespread in the 1950s. In turn, this development has led to progress in comfort, personal hygiene and privacy, and better regulation of infectious organisms in institutions; however, it has also made it more difficult for families to visit their sick relatives, and as a consequence, has led to an increase in solitary deaths in hospital (Nguyen, 2013, p. 1). The management of death has become more professional, and the observance of its rituals more restricted; the handling of corpses and funerals has become the exclusive province of undertakers, with children and more distantly-related friends and relatives often being excluded from participation in the obsequies (Nguyen, p. 1). The inability of the living to communicate with the dying noted by Elias (1985) and Stearns (1994), is becoming more pronounced.

As the twentieth century progressed, decaying and incontinent bodies became increasingly repugnant to us, necessitating their being kept hidden away. Patients admitted to hospices for symptom control but nevertheless, unable to avoid making messes, became humiliated by their loss of dignity and at times, their felt repulsiveness to relatives, and even to staff (Lawton, 1998). Since we now live longer and sometimes, with repellent and deteriorating conditions that medical science cannot mask, sequestration and sedation of terminally-ill individual patients – often at their own request – is not unusual. None of this is publicly acknowledged; this is apparent in a rather idealised online statement about palliative care, put forward by the Australian Department of Health:

> [It is] an approach to improve the quality of life of patients and their families facing the problems associated with life-threatening illness, through the prevention and relief of suffering by means of early

> identification and impeccable assessment and treatment of pain and other problems, physical, psychosocial and spiritual.
>
> (who.int)

In fact, the practice of sequestering certain patients, and indeed, of the whole gut-wrenching nature of a segment of end of life care, becomes apparent in the gap between the sometimes "terrible reality of deaths in the hospice" and, for example, "the glossed-up, distancing versions with calm patients demonstrating dignified acceptance of death" that are presented to the public (Hockey, 2007, p. 438). Open cancerous wounds and the incontinence of damaged organs are nobody's fault, but in our sanitised society, the expectation of their being repugnant to others renders them deeply shameful.

Sequestration as a function of our construction of social reality

American sociologists Berger and Luckman contend that:

> Society is built up by activity that expresses subjective meaning .... An adequate understanding of the 'reality *sui generis*' of society requires an inquiry into the manner in which this reality is constructed.
>
> (Berger & Luckman, 1966, p. 30)

As a corollary to this, they hold that although sometimes fragile, the social meanings of institutions provide their members with a sense of reality and identity. Hugh Willmott, an exponent of the hypothesis that our sequestration of death is symptomatic of our fear of it, suggests that the background to this fear can be found in our society's loss of religious belief: "Legitimations – notably, pre-modern religious beliefs – served to channel and assuage the transpersonal and existential significance of mortality" (Willmott, 2000, Death. So What?, p. 655). Indeed, now that established religion's capacity to infuse our lives with meaning has virtually disappeared, our fear of mortality has likely been much enhanced. Having once had an intelligible place in a religion-based interpretation of the meaning of life, death is becoming meaningless to us, an arbitrary termination of our ever onward and upward progress.

Accordingly, for some social theorists, the primary function of sequestration of the dead and dying is to facilitate our need to turn a blind eye to these reminders of our own ultimate destiny.

Sequestration as a psychosocial function of the fear of death

In their 1972 book, *The American view of death*, semantic scholars Dumont and Foss contend that, in order to retain our grasp on reality, we are obliged to accept that death is real, but at the same time, in order to go about our business with any sense of commitment, we deny its absolute power over how long we will live (as cited by Mellor & Shilling, 1993, p. 411). In response to this challenge to understand the human dilemma about mortality, theoretical rather than empirical sociological texts about human attitudes to death proliferated in the 1980s and 1990s; some of these are discussed below. British sociologists Stanley and Wise are critical of these texts on the grounds that as they enjoy 'canonical status', they are taken as presenting integrated ideas and facts about changing attitudes to dying rather than merely their authors' own arguments, unsupported by empirical research. In particular, they object to these theorists making the assumption that everyone deals with death in the same way (Stanley & Wise, 2011, pp. 949–950). Given the continuing lack of in-depth research into individual attitudes to death and dying up to now, however, they had little alternative.

The next section presents four of these theoretical contributions, three of which are focused on sequestration as a psychosocial expression of our fear of facing death and at the same time, a demonstration of our need to remain unaware of it. Writers discussed include Hugh Willmott (2000, *Death. So What?*), Anthony Giddens (1991, *Modernity and self-identity*), Philip Mellor and Chris Shilling (1993, *Modernity, self-identity and the sequestration of death*), and Liz Stanley and Sue Wise, who alone include two case studies (2011, *The sequestration thesis and the domestication of death*). Note that the analysis of the articles which follows does not attempt to give a comprehensive exposition of the authors' body of work, but focuses on those aspects which relate directly to the sequestration of death in modern society.

Hugh Willmott (2000): Sequestration and identification with the indestructible

Social theorists like Zygmunt Bauman hold that it is innate in humanity to see death as something negative, but to organisational analyst Hugh Willmott, our feeling of fear towards death is an artefact, a social product which has to be explained. He writes that he has seen no contribution to this issue in sociological studies; in a kind of dual-layered defence against mortality awareness, he finds that death's significance in the motivation of human conduct is itself sequestered and disregarded. For Willmott, this neglect is just another example of how death's existence is shunned; he believes that this is because death has the potential to render absurd and futile every project and institution that endows our lives with meaning and value. Therefore, the projects of contemporary society are all "conditional upon a suspension of our knowledge of mortality" (Willmott, 2000, p. 655). Acknowledging that there is a resonance between symbolic death – the experience of losing one's sense of self-identity – and physical death, Willmott contends that nevertheless, they are not coterminous. Rather, he holds that it is humanity which conflates the two and having done so, disavows threats to both together by keeping up a business-as-usual sense of what is real, and the pursuit of life-enhancing activities.

Amongst other social theorists, Willmott attributes our supposed ever-unassuaged, existential anxiety about our mortality in part to our having "debunked the idea of an afterlife" (p. 651). As a consequence, he argues, when death approaches, we find ourselves exposed to an awareness of the insignificant nature of the projects which, rather than assessing them for their existential value, we have depended upon for our sense of immortal self-identity. Accordingly, when death is in the offing, we are left with an overwhelming sense of confusion and insignificance, because it confronts us with "the projected loss of what we (commonsensically) know or believe ourselves to be: the socially-constructed sense of self-identity, that arises simultaneously with participation in modern institutions" (Willmott, 2000, p. 658). For Bauman (1992), we fear death because we believe that death equates with the chaos we imagine underlies the vulnerable social institutions that we have created to stave it off; in death, we fear the loss of this ordered, comprehensible world, and a resultant descent into eternal pandemonium. Willmott, however, holds the obverse view; for him, anomic terror is aroused in us by the prospect of symbolic death or the loss of our own self-identity, not of the constructed world. Unlike Bauman, he believes that institutions have an authentic function in our society, which is independent of our use of them as a prop for our sense of ontological security.

Willmott is not writing about persons; he is generalising about certain putative patterns of thought, and this creates a cohort of stereotypes, rather than individuals. Unlike the participants in the present study, Willmott's hypothetical population has not yet been faced with death but as construed, is intent upon avoiding it. His hypothesis that when threatened with personal death, people feel it as a terrifying threat to their sense of self-identity, fails to hold up when tested against data from the present investigation, as presented in Chapter 8, *Themes in the experience of dying*.

Anthony Giddens (1991): Sequestration and the protection of bodily integrity

Veteran British sociologist, Anthony Giddens, describes sequestration in modern society as the product of "increased control of internally-referential systems, operating not through discourse but institutional correlates, which remove aspects of living from day-today-life, with madness, criminality, sickness, death, sexuality being the key areas in which sequestration has become supreme" (Giddens, 1991, p. 161). Like Walter and Willmott, Giddens thinks that in modern society, there has been a reduction in the scope of the sacred and a loss of the communal in people's experience of death. He agrees with Willmott that, no longer able to rely on factors like location or ritual to define them, modern humanity must construct a sense of self-identity for themselves, and that this far-reaching social change is central to the endorsement of sequestration by society in general. However, the similarity of their views ends there.

Giddens identifies the human body – with all its processes, thoughts and feelings – rather than institutions, as integral to the project of developing one's self-identity; as a consequence, we find the presence of death disturbing in a social setting made up of reflexively-constructed, self-narratives centred on the body (Giddens, pp. 70–108). Accordingly, sequestration of the sick and dying offers society some security from the threat of unwanted encounters with damaged bodies and corpses, and therefore, some degree of ontological security. On the other hand, Giddens does not see this kind of sequestration as ultimately to society's advantage. He believes that, in thus escaping from contact with those we reject, the rest of society is the poorer, because it is being depleted by "the concealment … of certain crucial life experiences" (Giddens, 1991, p. 162).

In Giddens' view, institutional functions are also important in terms of the support they offer a society fearful of death. His view is closer to Bauman's than to Willmott's, but for Giddens, it is not the existence of orderly routines and institutions *per se* that protects society against chaos. Rather, it is the reassuring *process of routinisation* itself (Giddens' emphasis) that insulates individuals to some degree from the threat that death poses to them. Nevertheless, despite our best efforts to remain unaware of it, death continues to turn up; Giddens thinks that this is the reason that it is the subject of increasing public debate. In the final analysis, for Giddens, the process of dying is seen as the incipient loss of the control which alone ensures our security: "Death is unintelligible exactly because it is the point zero at which control lapses" (Giddens, 1991, p. 203).

Giddens deals in generalities – like his contemporaries, he lacks the information needed to discuss individual differences in attitudes to death – but he does recognise that this is a gap in sociological research. Unlike Willmott, for whom arguably, persons are represented as a kind of hypothetical construct, for Giddens, persons are aware and thinking individuals. As Giddens sees us, rather than being merely passive entities in a set of pre-ordained, scripted moves, we are real human beings, each struggling to find a way to relate to the society in which we find ourselves living.

Philip Mellor and Chris Shilling (1993): Sequestration and the shrinkage of the sacred

American social and religious theorists, Philip Mellor and Chris Shilling, also aim to provide a theoretical overview of the relationship between self-identity and the structuring of death in contemporary society. The primary issue for them is that, as compared with times of widespread religious observance, we are now thrown back on ourselves to find meaning in life and death; as a result, we find ourselves subject to "reality-threatening ontological and existential anxieties", with no strategies for facing our mortality (Mellor & Shilling, 1993, p. 423). At the same time, they find that there is a decrease in the public, or community space given to death and the dying, and a shrinkage of the sacred; there has been a "radical privatisation of the organisation of death" (Mellor & Shilling, 1993, p. 414). They argue that death is now a private and hidden experience – typically occurring in isolation in hospital – contending that this is because the visible dying have become a threat to people's egotistical self-identities. As they see it, "contemporary cosmic narcissism rejects traditional religious beliefs" because religious doctrines do not support the current focus on "praying for one's own self-interest and eternal survival" (Mellor & Shilling, 1993, p. 424). Further, they hold that, where once we reserved communal reverence for a deity external to, and far above ourselves, people now treat their own bodies as vessels of the sacred and immortal. This is evident in our devotion to ourselves, to our "self-care", to investing in "alternative healing systems" and pursuing "growth and self-actualisation" (pp. 423–424). According to Mellor and Shilling, however, this constant preoccupation with ourselves will be to no avail; in their view, given that there is no longer a language for working through its ontological reality, repeated experiences of death as meaningless will in time reveal to us "the futility of these activities" (p. 424).

For Mellor and Shilling, life in high modernity has led directly to sequestration, to a strengthening of boundaries between living and dying bodies, and in particular, to a diminution of space occupied by the sacred. They define the sacred as "set apart from the profanity of day-to-day life, and imbued with a special self-transcending significance", and argue that "it ... satiates human anxiety about meaning and order" (p. 429). Finding meaning in life is not merely a cognitive issue; for them, a significant aspect of the loss of religion in modernity is the deconstruction of value systems, along with their rituals, and bodily referents and practices.

Most writers discussing their views on the connection between sequestration and death in modernity refer to the disruptive part played in it by the passing of traditional religious observance. However, only Mellor and Shilling write in tones of such righteous anger about it, particularly about people withdrawing reverence from the deities of the past and trying instead, to find the sacred within themselves, or in other things or people. Humankind seems always to have been disposed to seek eternal truth, although the object to be venerated as its repository has varied from one culture or era to another. Generally, the trend has been to search for the sacred in some deified other or others and to Mellor and Shilling, there seems to be a kind of lese-majesté attached to locating it within ourselves. And yet, in contemporary society, religious belief has not so much ceased as changed; apart from the self-care and self-actualisation pursuits and followerships of various gurus in the field, many people value the pursuit of the non-sectarian spiritual, new religious groups are springing up, and some ancient beliefs like Islam and Buddhism have developed a renewed appeal. In modernity, rather than being lost, the capacity for reverence may be moving away from the dogmas of the recent past towards a synthesis of the old with the new. According to Elias (1985), for example, if not in terms of an afterlife for those who have no such expectation, death can still be made meaningful in the way the life that is ending is celebrated (p. 62). Ways in which death can be meaningfully celebrated, or an appropriate *ars moriendi* created, are discussed in Chapter 8, *Themes in the experience of dying.*

Arguably, humanity is on the move towards a future which will be as different from its receding past as now-forgotten earlier eras were from theirs; change is taking place in many of our practices and values. As seen in the next section, according to Stanley and Wise, rather than signalling our failure to grasp the conflict with which death faces us, or to respond constructively to what the dying need from us, sequestration may play a crucial part in our acceptance of the transition from what we are now to what we must all become.

Liz Stanley and Sue Wise (2011): Sequestration is necessary to creative adaptation

Until the nineteenth century, deaths occurred mainly in the domestic space; after that, they were increasingly drawn into a civil-institutional context and thereafter, the dying were sequestered in hospitals, nursing homes and once dead, in funeral parlours. For British sociologists Stanley and Wise (2011), Elias' (1985) view that sequestration of death and the dying did not replace domestic figuration, but occurred alongside its continued importance, holds the key to understanding what is taking place. They reject the idea of "a juggernaut of sequestration" and claim that in its present form, "the domestication of death" involves a complex set of sometimes contradictory processes – which include those of sequestration – and is "experienced and mediated through the nexus of domestic configuration" (Stanley &Wise, 2011, p. 948). Unlike many theorists about the meaning of sequestration, Elias works from empirical evidence; Stanley and Wise agree with his contention that our mutually-oriented interdependencies are the nexus of domestic figuration (p. 951). In their view, exploring the dynamics of groups of people in figurational terms rather than individualistic ones enables us to allow modernity's sequestration processes to remain at the core, while at the same time, we continue to investigate changing patterns of social relations at local, especially family levels.

According to Elias (as cited in Stanley & Wise, 2011, p. 951), it is true that "states of fear and terror of death" do continue, in both individual and institutional contexts, to characterise societies which feature sequestration. In an exploratory move forward from this point, however, Stanley and Wise investigate the possibility that, rather than being an end in itself, sequestration re presents a stage in our society's eventual adaptation to death and dying. Given that Elias' notion of domestic figuration includes both the home and its occupants and the network of relationships around it, they argue that, if taken together, these constitute the familiar everyday setting through which, people bring what is 'out there' and 'in here' together. Thus, in the process essential to all adaptation, what is 'other' is gradually made 'our own'. Even when, like death, the 'other' is challenging or upsetting, a 'taming' or 'ritualising' process crucial to domesticating the interaction of the known with the ineffable unknown can take place; this is a continuous operation, involving the constant rethinking of binary notions of public and private (Stanley & Wise, 1993, p. 953).

In fact, the actual process may involve quite commonplace moves, and it is when activities once perceived as opposites are integrated that a new domestic ritual can evolve. Such a process can occur even at the major transitional point when a family member is dying; continuing domestic routines go on alongside events experienced by the family as traumatic and threatening. Under these conditions, ordinary events can acquire a magical quality because in that particular situation, they are experienced as transgressive of the ordinary. For example, an elderly comatose woman was dying slowly in hospital from a sudden cerebral haemorrhage which, to the consternation of the family, had overtaken her when they were out and she was alone. As she had been fastidious about her appearance, a ritual developed in which relatives would gently wash her face and comb her hair; they were convinced that before she died, she had begun to look quite pretty and perhaps, at some level, appreciated their efforts to care for her. Further examples of this kind of adaptation to a loved one's dying, and its sometimes transformative effects on everyone involved, are seen in the *ars moriendi* rituals described in Chapter 8, *Themes in the experience of dying*. According to Stanley and Wise, "Such things ... produce an environment which re-establishes notions of order, and thereby helps deal with the circumstances which occasioned the need for them" (p. 954).

Although in modernity, sequestration and the civil-institutional sphere regulate many aspects of life, Stanley and Wise hold that sequestration does not prevent private moments between family members, or supersede public ritualised activities like funerals and memorial services, which include the relatives. Indeed, some new practices have appeared, and are becoming accepted by institutions and families alike. For example, in many hospitals nowadays, families can virtually 'camp out' in the hospital room, talk and minister to, and generally accompany a dying member for days prior to their death. In fact, far from excluding it, sequestration actually requires the domestic figuration to do many such indispensable parts of its work – for example, informing people of the death, and organising the disposal of the body. Some long-established rituals like viewing still persist, and some new ones have begun, like roadside shrines to remember accident victims, and spontaneous memorials to grieve the loss of public figures; in fact, rituals which enable people to relate to the dead and dying as familiar, knowable and mourned, are becoming more widespread and popular. Stanley and Wise conclude: "The ultimate challenge is to embrace the ineffable, the immateriality of what death 'is'" (p. 959). Sequestration both mediates and runs alongside an adaptation to a new phase in which, rather than trying to reject change and regress to previous times, we strive to create new rituals, new language and new frameworks of what is valuable or to be revered. Once unfamiliar ways of doing and seeing things – perhaps, even finding dying an acceptable, even though an absolute, ending to a life – can eventually become familiar, even trusted.

The section which follows examines the organisational and operational form of sequestration of the dying, usually within an institution.

Sequestration as the separation of the dying from the living

The writers presented in this section include Julia Lawton (1998, *Contemporary hospice care: The sequestration of the unbounded body and 'dirty dying'*), Katherine Froggatt (2001, *Life and death in English nursing homes: Sequestration or transition?*), Norbert Elias (1985, *The loneliness of the dying*) and Clive Seale (1995, *Dying alone*).

Julia Lawton's Contemporary hospice care and Katherine Froggatt's Life and death in English nursing homes

Lawton's and Froggatt's papers cover related areas of sequestration practices in healthcare institutions; therefore, they are discussed together.

Julia Lawton (1998): Sequestration: A response to unbearable dying

British medical sociologist Julia Lawton's 1998 article, based on her ten months as a participant-researcher in an English hospice, shocked many when it was first published. In contrast with modern society's ideals that hospice care provides living personhood and a hygienic, somatically-bound body, Lawton contends that the sequestered dying that she saw taking place in hospices provides rather for a kind of decaying, disintegrating body that in Western society, is not tolerated anywhere else. In case Lawton's work may seem outdated, this is not a problem that has by now been made to go away. According to social researcher Kate Woodthorpe's 2010 review of Lawton's article, nothing had changed. And today, by their very nature, contemporary extensions of life – despite sometimes dreadful symptoms and featuring 'heroic' treatments – seem likely to make accommodation of the kind of suffering described by Lawton more, rather than less necessary.

As one of her illustrations, Lawton presents Annie, a sixty-seven year-old woman who requested admission for palliative care but especially, for symptom control. She had developed an untreatable pelvic cancer, which had spread rapidly and was causing bouts of malodourous incontinence at home, in front of her husband and adult son. Once admitted, she rapidly developed a recto-vaginal fistula, which led to reeking urine and faeces pouring out of the same passage, covering her up to her shoulders in her bed; its stench penetrated the whole building, drifting beyond the front door. At this stage, the nurses described Annie as "rotting down below". Feeling utterly humiliated, she insisted that her attentive husband stop visiting and finally, asked to be sedated and moved to a side room, where she withdrew into silence. Six weeks after being admitted, she died, with no family present.

With such uncontrollable conditions, patients were obliged to remain in the hospice until they died; they invariably disengaged, stopped talking, eating and drinking, and stared into space. The patient's sense of self seemed to have 'gone', with some seeking a hastened death; none ever recovered. According to Lawton, Annie's was far from an isolated case; Lawton calls conditions like hers "having unbounded bodies" (Lawton, 1998, p. 128–9).

Lawton argues that hospices in this instance serve as "fringe-liminal" spaces, holding these in effect "non-persons" buffered between two worlds, and that such sequestering and marginalising practices are "culturally and historically specific to bodily unboundedness" (p. 132). From her account, it seems that the unbounded also sequester themselves, first by leaving home to seek substitute bodily boundaries in hospices and then, because they are so repugnant both to others and to themselves, by undergoing a total evacuation of their sense of self and social identity from their intolerable bodies. Trapped in this nightmare scenario, the individual has no way of processing or influencing what is happening to them, and no other escape route. Moreover, according to Lawton, there can be no reprieve; in order for mainstream society to feel secure in the belief that their world and in particular, they themselves, are reliably hygienic, sanitised and somatically-bounded, sequestration can never be abandoned (Lawton, 1998, p. 139).

Katherine Froggatt (2001): Sequestration: A transitional state between two polarities

Like Lawton, basing her observations on many hours as a participant-researcher, British nursing academic, Katherine Froggatt, concluded that at least for nursing home residents, sequestration did not separate the living from the dying, but was rather "the creation of transitional states between two polarities" (Froggatt, 2001, p. 320). For Froggatt, whether the institution in question was a hospice, residential care facility or nursing home, the organisation of space and boundaries within them necessarily developed differently to accommodate the significant variations in their populations. For example, hospice residents' entry criteria usually required that their dying trajectory be short term and predictable, whereas the dying trajectories of nursing home residents were often unpredictable, because they were not clearly defined. Patterns of life in the two institutions, and staff systems of working with their patients, differed significantly.

According to Froggatt, making the basic distinction to set the dying apart from the living in an older population requires expertise, and is often problematic for both staff and the residents themselves; identifying the dying amongst the frail elderly is much less straightforward than it is with younger people.

Many of the elderly have chronic diseases, and the very old often have states of non-specific gradual deterioration; neither of these conditions is subject to a terminal diagnosis or to its sufferers being classed as dying. Death from general deterioration is the least understood of deaths, and may take place over months or even years; staff called it "failing", or "being poorly", and found that in these circumstances, distinguishing the living from the dying was often not possible (Froggatt, 2001, p. 325). For Froggatt, it was how the patients progressed through the transitional state of the living-dying interval that was relevant to working with them, rather than absolute categories of life and death.

Given the evidence, Froggatt concludes that sequestration took place spontaneously in response to the exigencies of nursing home life, rather than being imposed upon it. Firstly, as "poorly" patients deteriorated, they began to withdraw to quiet corners or to their rooms; some of them developed some unboundedness and would go for long spells with staff to bathrooms. Secondly, the boundaries were very marked in the public spaces – the alert and capable spontaneously gathered in one area, and the less alert or confused in another. As Froggatt observes, the part played by the institution in this pattern of sequestration was to provide possibilities for transitional states between living and dying, which allowed the patients to come and go for months between well and unwell. Until death came, there was no need for permanent separations. In this instance, sequestration occurred naturally, even supportively, alongside the fluctuations of patients' well-being, and appeared neither distressing nor stigmatising to them. In this respect, Froggatt's account of her patients' use of the institution's spaces to manage a gradual adaptation to their deteriorating health, is not unlike Stanley and Wise's description of the function of domestic figurational movements in adapting to new and alarming events in the outside world.

Mellor and Shilling suggest that, whether societal, or within institutions, sequestration's ultimate aim is to strengthen boundaries to prevent the impingement of sickness and death on the everyday life of the rest of society (Mellor & Shilling, 1993, p. 320). Lawton's conclusion was more specific; that since mainstream society needed to feel secure in the belief that their world was safely hygienic, sanitised and somatically-bounded, unbounded bodies must be kept sequestered (Lawton, 1998, p. 139). By contrast, however, although like Lawton, and unlike Mellor and Shilling, her conclusions were based on grounded evidence and obtained within a similar time-frame, Froggatt's experience of sequestration was at odds with that of her colleagues. For her, at least within nursing homes, the organisation of space and setting of boundaries was responsive to the needs of the patient groups and facilitative of the staff's interactions with them. Now, unlike all the other writers on the subject of sequestration, Froggatt was an experienced nurse; to her, the sights, smells and sounds of the very ill were part of her everyday duty of care, while for the those like the more academic Lawton, such experiences could well be shocking, and their impact, correspondingly disturbing.

Although it may seem so to us, our contemporary society's profound aversion to being close to repellent scenes of sickness and death is not innate; it is a product of our society's learnt fear and repugnance towards a cohort of human misery. To some degree, this attitude can be seen to represent a hygiene survival kit, but it may also suggest that in our image of ourselves, we are becoming less robust, and more inclined to expect protection from unpleasant realities. As both Elias (1985) and Giddens (1991) intimated that it would, some once-present ability to handle life's tougher attributes seems to be leaching out of us through their being removed from our experience. This could be problematic; sheltering ourselves from life's nastier aspects could confirm our image of ourselves as unable to face the ugly side of things, and where adaptation is needed, trap us instead in a vicious cycle of avoidance.

Norbert Elias (1985): Sequestration and shameful dying

Elias defines sequestration as "the tacit isolation of the ageing and dying from their community of the living, with the gradual cooling of their relationships to people to whom they are attached, the separation from human beings in general, who gave them meaning and security" (Elias, 1985, p. 2). In his view, the sequestration of the dying occurs relatively early in advanced societies and since it has the power to isolate us from each other, our societies will be the weaker for it. Seeing sequestration as a learnt, rather than an innate behaviour, he believes that it shows how the living in our societies increasingly fail to identify with ageing and dying. An aspect of the comprehensive "civilising spurt" which takes away power and respect from the elderly and dying, it creates around them a climate of shame, repugnance and embarrassment (Elias, 1985, p. 11). For him, this kind of sequestration represents more than an unfortunate if limited failure of compassion; the aversion expressed towards the old and the sick is, to him, a creeping social disease which is spreading to include many other groups, and may eventually leave us all distrustful of intimacy with or dependence on each other.

Humanity's multi-faceted sequestration activities are not seen by Elias as defensive only against a fear of death or illness. Rather, he sees sequestration behaviours as part of a general attempt on our part to achieve control over everything – or everyone – "rather than developing our own more positive communal life" (Elias, 1985, p. 81). Giddens had experienced a similar insight; he thought that humanity feared dying because it represented a loss of the control over events that we are convinced alone ensures our security (Giddens, 1991, p. 203). For Willmott, Mellor and Shilling, and Lawton, on the other hand, sequestration is imposed specifically in the service of our secularised society's need to remain unaware of death and of terrible ways to die. In yet another take on the matter, for Stanley and Wise, and for Froggatt, creative sequestration can promote flexibly organised care of the frail and dying, and enable the adaptation to challenging circumstances that will be needed for us to explore better targeted ways of meeting their needs.

Clive Seale (1995): Sequestration as security against dying alone

Data from friends and relatives of 149 people who had died alone formed the basis of research carried out by British medical sociologist, Clive Seale. Unlike the previous writers – who viewed it as a necessary, or even negative factor in the management of the frail elderly – Seale's researches have inclined him to regard sequestration in hospitals, for example, as a positive phenomenon, because it provides them with a place of safety.

From the accounts of the lone deaths at home in his data, he discovered the importance to his respondents of having an opportunity for "*resurrective practice*" (p. 378, his emphasis). He contends that: "[all our] hopes rest on the security that comes from successful claims to membership of a caring community", such as concerned body corporates, or carers' groups (p. 378). The majority of his respondents were neighbours or friends of the deceased; they thought that the often unexpected deaths alone at home were regrettable, and wished that they had been there. Seale believes that his findings illustrate the threat posed by the lone death to the widely-shared ideal of being able to help and accompany the dying: an ideal of the caring community which offers some solace to many in our frequently fragmented contemporary society. Of course, dying alone is not restricted to those who live alone; people can die unaccompanied at home when everyone else is asleep or out, or in hospital, when staff and family are not present. For Seale, as for Stanley and Wise (2011, p. 948), there is no monolithic "juggernaut of sequestration"; society is made up of multiple localities and their inhabitants, and communal involvement in people's dying is still extensive. Indeed, Seale claims that, for as long as people are concerned with being members of a caring community which deems them "worthy of a network of love and trust", it will always be so (1995, p. 389).

Rather against the tide of opinion, Seale argues that the maintenance of emotional order, basic functions, and regulation of the dying trajectory, are all best served by the hospitalisation of the dying. He contends that in modern times, a professionalised death in hospital may be preferable to death at home, where one may still die alone, and potentially beyond medical support or resurrective practice. Certainly, his respondents believed that dying alone at home was a bigger threat to the image of a caring community than dying alone in hospital was. Moreover, a study by Macartney, Broom, Kirby, Good and Adams of how patients with acute palliative care needs experienced different locales of care, and how this impacted on their understanding of dying, found that although dying at home was highly rated by patients, there was remarkably little resistance in practice to their having to abandon this desire, and go to hospital or to a hospice (Macartney et al., 2016, para 5). Contending that any established death rites can support the working through of mourning for a death, Seale refers to the anthropologist Loring Danforth's suggestion (1982, as cited in Seale, p. 389), that such "reality-sustaining rites" allow the bereaved to continue the conversation with the deceased and then, gradually to let it go, and begin new conversations.

Mellor and Shilling (1993) contend that a significant aspect of the loss of religion in modernity is the deconstruction of value systems, but they make no mention of what, if anything, might fill the resultant void. Similarly, Elias claims that compassion for the sick and the elderly is actually disappearing. On the other hand, if Seale is right, and given that more and more people now live in apartment blocks and outlying suburban precincts, perhaps this groundswell of caring communities will continue to grow, and to sustain their members. Arguably, such values do not belong only to religious believers or previous generations; rather, they are a fundamental characteristic of all socialised human beings.

Summing up the debate

Due to the degree of medicalisation of our society's end of life care, the sequestration of a number of chronically-ill and frail elderly people is inevitable; for some commentators, no further explanation of sequestration is needed. For others, however, such practices are not merely responses to perceived need; rather, they are expressions of our wish to remain unaware of our mortality and vulnerability to grave illness. In disagreement with this view, however, some sociologists argue that sequestration can be understood as an essential step in adaptation to change by permitting the gradual exploration of the unknown and thus, the evolution of new patterns of care. Accordingly, in response to changing patterns of living and working, and even if we do still avoid thinking about death and the ravages of dying, we will continue to form caring communities prepared to accept responsibility for our sick and dying members.

Summary of chapter

While difficulties for us in thinking about our own death do exist, it has been argued that, taken gradually, and including children, we can resist thus being silenced, and become more accustomed to expressing our understanding of what death means to us. On the other hand, whether because it is a taboo subject, or merely bad manners to raise the subject of personal death, some commentators argue that death is not talked about because the unwritten rules of everyday conversation forbid it. It is possible, however, that change is in the air, and that for people of all ages, a desire for more openness on the subject is growing. The chapter ends with a study of sequestration of the dead and dying; whether this is primarily a symptom of our wish to be shielded from this area of human experience, or whether it is a part of how we can best adapt to it, remains a matter of debate. Perhaps in the vicissitudes of the changes taking place at present in our attitudes to death and dying, our sequestration practices include something of both.

Next follows Chapter 3, Thanatology: Reflections on the meaning of death. The term 'my death' represents our understanding of what the experience of death is like and therefore, is as much a social construct as a biological fact. Based on this view, a history is given of the changes in our attitudes to our own death from antiquity to the present. Special emphasis is given to the upsurge in death studies, or thanatology, in the twentieth century. A philosophical discussion of whether or not death does us harm ends the chapter.

References

Ballatt, J., & Campling, P. (2011). *Intelligent kindness: Reforming the culture of healthcare*. London: RCPsych Publications.

Bartalos, M. (2008). *Speaking of death: America's new sense of mortality*. Westport, CT: Praeger Publishers.

Bauman, Z. (1992). *Mortality, immortality and other life strategies*. Palo Alto, CA: Stanford University Press.

BBC News. (2018, February 26). Call to end 'taboo' of talking about death. *BBC News Health Report*. Retrieved from https://www.bbc.com/news/health-43169284

Becker, E. (1973). *The denial of death*. New York: Free Press.

Behrendt, K. (2010). A special way of being afraid. *Philosophical Psychology, 23*(5), 669–682. doi: 10.1080/09515089.2010.514573

Berger, P., & Luckman, T. (1966). *The social construction of reality*. New York: Anchor Press.

Caughlin, J. P., Mikucki-Enyart, S. L., Middleton, A. V., Stone, A. M., & Brown, L. E. (2011). Being open without talking about it: A rhetorical/normative approach to understanding topic avoidance in families after a lung cancer diagnosis. *Communication Monographs, 78*(4), 409–436. doi: 10.1080/03637751.2011.618141

Clarke, L. H., Korotchenko, A., & Bundon, A. (2012). 'The calendar is just about up': Older adults with multiple chronic conditions reflect on death and dying. *Ageing and Society, 32*(8), 1399–1417. Retrieved from https://www.ncbi.nlm.nih.gov/pubmed/24976657

Corke, C. (2018). *Letting go: How to plan for a good death*. London and Brunswick, Melbourne: Scribe Books.

Corke, C., & Hillman, K. (2018, July 28). *How to achieve a good death* [Interview with Geraldine Doogue, Radio National Saturday Extra]. Retrieved from http://www.abc.net.au/radionational/programs/saturdayextra/what-is-a-good-death/1C

Davis-Berman, J. (2011). Conversations about death: Talking to residents in independent, assisted, and long-term care settings. *Journal of Applied Gerontology, 30*(3), 353–369. doi: 10.1177/0733464810367637

De Raedt, R., Koster, E. H., & Ryckewaert, R. (2013). Aging and attentional bias for death-related and general threat-related information: Less avoidance in older as compared with middle-aged adults. *Journals of Gerontology: Series B: Psychological Sciences and Social Sciences, 68*(1), 41–48. doi: 10.1093/geronb/gbs047

Di Masi, F. (2004). *Making death thinkable*. London: Free Association Books.

Elias, N. (1985). *The loneliness of the dying*. E. Jephcott (Trans.). Oxford: Basil Blackwell Ltd.

Feifel, H. (1959). *The meaning of death*. London and New York: McGraw Hill Book Company

Froggatt, K. (2001). Life and death in English nursing homes: Sequestration or transition? *Ageing and Society, 21*, 319–332. doi: 10.1017/S0144686X0100825X

Gamliel, T. (2008). The macabre style: Death attitudes of old-age residents in Israel. *Ethos, Journal for the Society of Psychological Anthropology*. Retrieved from https://doi.org/10.1525/eth.2003.31.4.495

Gavin, W. J. (1995). *Cuttin' the body loose: Historical, biological, and personal approaches to death and dying*. Philadelphia, PA: Temple University Press.

Giddens, A. (1991). *Modernity and self-identity*. Stanford, CA: Stanford University Press.

Gorer, G. (1994). The pornography of death. In J. B. Williamson & E. S. Schneiderman (Eds.), *Death: Current Perspectives* (4th ed., pp. 73–77). Palo Alto: Mayfield Publishing Company.

Henig, R. M. (2005, August 7). Will we ever arrive at a good death? *The New York Times Magazine*, pp. 26–35. Retrieved from http://www.nytimes.com/2005/08/07/magazine/07DYINGL.html?pagewanted=all=&_r=0

Hockey, J. (2007). Closing in on death? Reflections on research and researchers in the field of death and dying. *Health Sociology Review, 16*(5), 436–446. doi: 10.5172/hesr.2007

Howarth, G. (2007a). *Death and dying: A sociological introduction*. Cambridge: Polity.

Kellehear, A. (2014). *The inner life of the dying person*. New York & Chichester: Columbia University Press.

Lawton, J. (1998). Contemporary hospice care: The sequestration of the unbounded body and 'dirty dying'. *Sociology of Health and Illness, 20*(2), 121–143. doi: 10.1111/1467–9566.00094

MacArtney, J., Broom, A., Kirby, E., Good., P., Wootton, J., & Adams, J. (2016). Locating care at the end of life: Burden, vulnerability, and the practical accomplishment of dying. *Sociology of Health and Illness, 38*(3), 479–492. doi: 10.1111/1467–9566.12375

Marie Curie Hospice, UK. (2017, October 19). Help us break the taboo around death. *Marie Curie blog, 2017*. Retrieved from mariecurie.org.uk/blog/taboo-death/167432

Mellor, P., & Shilling, C. (1993). Modernity, self-identity and the sequestration of death. *Sociology, 27*(3), 411–431. doi: 10.1177/0038038593027003005

Nguyen, T. (2013, September 29). Is death and dying now a "sequestrated" experience? *Society of Health Group Presentation, Term 1*. Retrieved from https://prezi.com/n7gon3sekrls/socy-health-group-presentation-term-1-is-death-and-dying-now-a-sequestrated-experience-in-latep/

News.com.au. (2018, May 25). Death Class: QLD schools encouraged to implement lessons about mortality. *Parenting – school life*. Retrieved from https://www.news.com.au/lifestyle/parenting/schools-life-death-class-qld-schools-encouraged-implement-lessons-about-mortality/news-story/2406b9aae78ebc483d10be655f093a2f

Palliative Care Australia (2013). *Election platform*. Retrieved 15/12/13 from http://www.palliativecare.org.au/Portals/46/Election%202007/Election/202013/PCA%20 Election20Statements.pdf

Parker, M. (2011, November 25). Body or soul: Why we don't talk about death and dying. *The Conversation*. Retrieved from https://the conversation.com/body-or-soul-why-we-dont-talk-about-death-and-dying-4354
Seale, C. (1995). Dying alone. *Sociology of Health and Illness, 17*(3), 376–392. Retrieved from https://onlinelibrary.wiley.com/doi/abs/10.1111/1467-9566.ep10933327
Seale, C. (1998). *Constructing death: The sociology of dying and bereavement*. Cambridge: Cambridge University Press.
Shewmon, D. A. (2010). Constructing the death elephant: A synthetic paradigm shift for the definition, criteria and tests for death. *Journal of Medicine and Philosophy, 35*(3), 256–298. doi: 10.1093/jmp/jhq022
Stanley, L., & Wise, S. (2011). The domestication of death: The sequestration thesis and domestic figuration. *Sociology, 45*(6), 947–962. doi: 10.1177/0038038511416153
Stearns, P. J. (1994). *American cool: Constructing a twentieth century emotional style*. New York: NYU Press.
Troyer, J. (2014, April 10). Death isn't taboo, we're just not encouraged to talk about it. *The Conversation*. Retrieved from https://theconversation.com/death-isn't-taboo-were-just-not-encouraged-to-talk-about-it-25001
Walter, T. (1991). Modern death: Taboo or not taboo? *Sociology, 25*(2), 293–310. doi: 10.1177/0038038591025002009
Whitman, M. (2019, February 26). The taboo of death. *Psychology Today*. Retrieved from https://www.psychologytoday.com/au/blog/sense-time/201902/the-taboo-death
Willmott, H. (2000). Death. So what? Sociology, sequestration and emancipation. *The Sociological Review, 48*(4), 649–665. Retrieved from https://onlinelibrary.wiley.com/doi/abs/10.1111/1467–954X.00237

3 Thanatology

Reflections on the meaning of death

Introduction: The study of death as a social construct

Thanatology is the scientific study of death, and the losses resulting from it. It investigates what happens to us physically when we die, as well as death's wider psychological and social attributes. It has many aspects, some of which are discussed in what follows.

The chapter opens with a history of our attitudes towards personal death through the ages, an account intended to provide not just a chronicle of events but also, to show how our understanding of the term 'my death' has evolved. Usually thought of as having an invariant meaning, the term 'my death' actually represents our understanding of what the experience of death is like and therefore, is as much a social construct as a biological event. As a consequence, what our death means to us subjectively has changed a great deal over the last two millennia. Socio-economic movements which have influenced our attitudes include the end of feudalism and the development of trade and commerce in the Middle Ages, improvements in public sanitation and in living standards generally during the Industrial Revolution, and with the secularisation of the body following the Enlightenment, the massive advances in medical knowledge of the twentieth century, accompanied by a surge in thanatological writing and research.

The chapter is divided into three parts, as follows:

Part I. From antiquity to the twentieth century: How our attitudes to death have changed
Part II. The twentieth century: The rise of thanatology
Part III. Philosophical opinion on death, ancient and modern: Does death cause us harm?

Part I. From antiquity to the twentieth century: How our attitudes to death have changed

Much of the information recorded here about historical attitudes towards death over the last two millennia, and some of its interpretation, is taken from Philippe Aries' 1974 account, *Western attitudes toward death from the*

DOI: 10.4324/9781003392088-3

Middle Ages to the present. Due to its research into a wide range of sources and to the detailed nature of its reporting, this work is acknowledged as the leading text of its genre. It has also generated criticism, however, and in the interests of providing a balanced account, some discussion of this debate is included.

Over the centuries, popular beliefs about life and death have undergone major changes, with significant implications for attitudes towards personal death. From societies dominated by a rigidly hierarchical agricultural economy with systems of belief framed by canon law and feudal custom, our societies are now largely governed through the secular authority of the state. As historian Chris Gilleard defines it, daily life in advanced societies is subject to the conditions of complex mercantile economies, characterised by dealings of an increasingly impersonal and technologically-controlled kind (Gilleard, 2002). Despite our awareness of these sweeping changes, we may assume that dying is such an archetypal experience that our attitude to it must have always been the same, but in fact, over the last two millennia, the way we see personal death has changed radically. A summary of the history of our attitudes toward death up to and including the nineteenth century follows:

- The first millennium: Primitive societies
- Toward the Middle Ages: Late first millennium to late eleventh century
- The Middle Ages: Late eleventh to sixteenth centuries
- The Enlightenment and the Industrial Revolution: Seventeenth to nineteenth centuries

The first millennium: Primitive societies

Historian Philippe Aries characterises the process of death and dying in this period as "tamed death" (Aries, 1974, p. 2). Disease was often rapidly fatal and most people knew when death was imminent. Dying was a community event, a public ritual carried out in the midst of the surrounding life; it was organised by the sick individual as a calming rite, to be performed in the bedchamber in the presence of helpers and mourners (Aries, 1974). Since the church was regarded as the final authority on life and death, dying took place according to a prescribed ritual. First, preparation for death required the individual to ask for forgiveness for himself, grant it to others where appropriate and then, to await death "lying down ... on his back so that his face is always turned toward heaven" with his arms folded across his chest so that "his body [was] ... forming a cross" (Aries, 1974, pp. 7–8). Fear of death in early societies was focused on death by untimely or unnatural agency, and on the deaths of significant others. In general, there seemed to be less concern felt about the individual's own death; like many other events, natural death was seen as just in the way of things (San Filippo, 2006). Following the death, however, because the dead took on a more alarming aspect, they were never mentioned again; feared by the living as potentially envious or vengeful, they were buried in cemeteries outside the towns, well away from its inhabitants (Aries, p. 15).

Until the eleventh and twelfth centuries, being cognisant of oneself as an individual with reflexive consciousness – someone who could be aware of having a personal life and death – would seldom have been found amongst ordinary folk (San Filippo, 2006, p. 6; Tucker, 2009, p. 1105); such a self-concept would have been limited to the privileged, to the clergy and the aristocracy. According to the seventh-century scholar the Venerable Bede, the general population's experience of life most resembled a single sparrow in flight:

> Entering at one door and leaving by another, while it is inside it is untouched by the wintry storm but this brief interval of calm is over in a moment, and it returns to the winter from whence it came ... Man's life is similar.
>
> (as cited in San Filippo, 2006, p. 7)

Men lived close to nature; "Familiarity with death [would have been] ... a form of acceptance of the order of nature" (Aries, 1974, p. 28). Together with the feudal system, the tenets of the church regarding the individual's expectations of entering heaven for righteousness, or hell as punishment for lacking it, constituted an effective means of social control.

Toward the Middle Ages: Late first millennium to late eleventh century

By the end of the first millennium, the unbridgeable divide between the living and the dead began to break down; cemeteries began to appear in the precincts of churches, and ossuaries and charnel houses proliferated on church premises. Now relating to the once-feared envious dead in a kind of macabre and appeasing intimacy, people gathered to socialise, dance and gamble, and even to trade all manner of merchandise alongside the charnel-houses (Aries, 1974, pp. 23–24). According to Aries, "the word 'cemetery' came to mean ... a cluster of houses enjoying certain fiscal or domanial privileges" (Aries, 1974, p. 23), and for those who could afford such prime real estate, a burial place close to the church was ardently sought. Side by side with booksellers and seamstresses, gravediggers would be reopening tombs and removing partly decomposed cadavers to permit a fresh burial (Aries, 1974, p. 25). This activity was well-tolerated; rather than providing the living with a disturbing glimpse of their future, perhaps their contact with corpses allowed them to congratulate themselves on still being alive.

The Middle Ages: Late eleventh to sixteenth centuries

During the period known as the Middle Ages, European society underwent the subtle and gradual but profound socio-cultural change of destabilisation, followed by the end of feudalism. Less dominated by a subsistence-based agricultural economy and moving towards a more complex mercantile economy, society began to develop a fluid and secular quality which relied for its governance on centres of economic exchange and the scientific thinking of the early Renaissance, rather than on the authority of the church and the upper class (Gilleard, 2002). With the breaking down of the enduring order of feudal society and the rise of a more materialistic and naturalistic understanding of demographic identification came a new order. But in the progress towards greater freedom for the individual, something was lost; without the protection of the church and the wealthy, special provision for the aged and frail came to an end (Gilleard, 2002). They have struggled to elicit adequate care ever since.

Side by side with this social transformation came a change in how religious iconography depicted salvation which, increasingly framed as an individual, rather than a mass event, became '*my* salvation' (Aries, 1974, p. 37). Tombs became more personalised, given to advertising the great deeds and hopes for immortality of their occupants. By contrast, in some European countries, images of worm-ridden corpses began to nudge the traditional recumbent knights to one side. Aries suggests that this more macabre style of iconography in the fourteenth century betrayed a bitter feeling of failure, "an anxiety at not sufficiently being" in life (Aries, 1974, p. 105) – an unease which has never ceased to trouble us.

There was another major change taking place; although "for more than a thousand years, people had been perfectly adapted to ... promiscuity between living and dead" (Aries, 1974, p. 25), during the sixteenth century, this kind of socialising was coming to an end: "We can see [developing] ... the deep-rooted refusal to link the end of the physical being with physical decay" (Aries, 1974, p. 33). In fact, the preoccupation of our contemporary society with sequestering the physical decay of death and dying was already beginning in the late fifteenth century, during which "a horror of physical death and decomposition [became] ... a familiar theme in ... [European] poetry" (Aries, 1974, p. 41). In contrast with the days of egalitarian socialising amongst corpses, decomposition was by now held to be symbolic of a man's "failure", a sign of his now profound and dismayed awareness of death and the fragility of life (Aries, 1974, p. 42). Following outbreaks of the Black Death from the fourteenth century on, this theme was further in evidence; representations of people and skeletons dancing together in the 'Dance of Death' imagery became common from the early fifteenth to the mid-sixteenth century. There was an iconoclastic aspect to these sketches; given that the lines of grisly frolickers showed popes, kings, labourers and children all taking part together, the social distinctions held to be important in life were being mocked in this portrayal of death as 'the great leveller'. Aries interprets these depictions of death as also "a sign of the love of life" (Aries, 1974, p. 45) – a passion whose poignancy was rendered even more intense by a dawning universal awareness of life's brevity.

Accordingly, as greater recognition and enjoyment of life flourished, individual living and being were the more celebrated, and identification with the community diminished. From the thirteenth to the fifteenth century, traditional church practices were being challenged by what mediaeval historian Jacob Burckhardt (1960) described as the new individualism, born of the promotion of individual talent during the Renaissance (as cited in Walter, 1991, p. 306). While death had previously been characterised by resignation and portrayed as a peaceful sleep ahead of a collective resurrection, the idea of judgement at death was now becoming highly personalised (Aries, 1974, p. 37). For the first time, the prospect of '*my* death' was capable of causing "a fear of the annihilation of the self", of one's existence simply vapourising (Tucker, 2009, p. 1105). Probably until then the prerogative of the educated and aristocratic classes, once it was represented to everyman as '*my own death*', the anticipation of his end could generate in anyone the fear of death which humanity has endured ever since. Erotico-macabre imagery depicting such events as "Death as Rapist" became common (Aries, 1974, p. 37); people were becoming outraged and repelled as well as disappointed that life must end in death.

Rather than being just one activity among the many happening in a household at any given time, dying began to occupy the central role in a solemn bedchamber ritual. By the end of the sixteenth century, death was no longer looked forward to as a chance to enter the afterlife but rather, rebelled against as the rupture of man's passionate attachment to things and creatures – the *temporalia* – won and loved during his lifetime. Accordingly, by now an abhorrent reminder of things to come, corporeal decay was banished from sight and gradually, the social activities in cemeteries were banned as irreverent (Aries, 1974).

On the other hand, the moment of death was for the first time thought of as providing a last chance for redemptive realisation by becoming the catalyst for an individual to finally grasp his own life-story, to discover the secret of his own individuality. According to Aries, by resisting despair at the ending of one's life and instead, seeking an understanding of one's own narrative from within the intense experience of facing one's death: "Death became the occasion when man was most able to reach an awareness of himself" (Aries, 1974, p. 52). Moreover, Aries believes that this hope has continued into our own time: "Since the early Middle Ages, man has come to see himself in his own death; he has discovered *la mort de soi*, one's own death" (Aries, 1974, p. 52). It is evident in the participant accounts in the present study that concern about the fate of the self remains of central importance to the dying.

Philosopher A. C. Grayling claims that the seventeenth century represented a turning point in human thought, forming a backdrop to the Renaissance and to the advances in scientific thinking of our modern age (Grayling, 2016, September 3, Interview, ABC Radio National). Even though there were reprisals in store for those who challenged the Church, the populace had begun to realise that no matter how powerful they were, groups like the

Church and the nobility did not possess a monopoly on knowledge. People were beginning to feel free to think things out for themselves, and rather than listening to their authoritarian rulers, they were turning for illumination to thinkers who could present empirical evidence or persuasive reasoning to support their opinions (Grayling, 2016).

The Enlightenment and the Industrial Revolution: Seventeenth to nineteenth centuries

Previously regarded as a time of anguished confrontation, personal death in the eighteenth century instead became romanticised. Often depicted in art and literature as ethereally lovely, dying and life after death were "believed to be beautiful peaceful experiences ... compared ... with the emergence of a butterfly from a cocoon" (San Filippo, 2006, p. 7). At the same time, however, now that family units were established based more on feeling and affection than on utility or convenience, their members had come to experience the death of loved ones as unbearably painful. With this significant change in relationship patterns, practices and attitudes surrounding death and mourning began to resemble more closely those which are familiar to us today. This newly romanticised view of death emphasised the possibility of "the immortality of the soul and of an eventual reunion of loved ones in the afterlife"; acquiring a burial place which could be held in perpetuity so that the living could come to commune with their lost loved ones became essential (San Filippo, 2006, p. 8). Nowadays, although visiting the graves of loved ones is not as common as it was in the twentieth century, it is still practised by some bereaved families. With these changes in public attitudes, by the nineteenth century the noxious cemeteries and charnel houses had gone, and properly kept cemeteries and memorials to the dead were allowed back into the cities (Aries, 1974); these are still respected by many as monuments to remembrance. Meanwhile, the new *ars moriendi* emerging in the nineteenth century emphasised the need to die peacefully and with dignity. Indeed, it was considered proper to keep the dying person unaware of, or at least, silent, about his condition, so that he would be able to retain his composure and above all, remain grateful; he should "[never] ... be indifferent to the efforts of those around him" (Gavin, 1995, p. 24). Nowadays, although a dignified and accepting death is still much sought-after, it is increasingly thought by contemporary palliative care professionals to be achieved not by keeping their true condition from the dying but rather, by encouraging them to feel and to express the full range of their feelings about it (Zimmerman, 2012, p. 217).

Due to the introduction of the use of steam, coal power and machine tools during the Industrial Revolution of the late eighteenth and nineteenth centuries, there was an unprecedented increase in the rate of production and distribution. Mass-producing factories replaced cottage industries, and the new production levels lifted everyone's living standards. Widespread improvements in sanitation, nourishment and health care saw a rise in quality of life, and an extension of life expectancy (Aries, 1974). Further, following the general acceptance in the seventeenth century of Descartes' theory that mind and body were made of different substances, science was no longer shackled by the idea of the sacredness of the body, as one with mind and spirit; it became possible for medical research "to take a giant leap forward" (Parker, 2011, p. 3). Indeed, until last century, investigation of mind and body had gone their separate ways, only fairly recently reuniting in modern 'combination' disciplines like neuropsychology.

By the late nineteenth century, a new intolerance of death had begun to seize those surrounding the dying; the old rituals remained, but were often accompanied by passionate expressions of sorrow and beseeching prayers as people became moved by the very idea of death. For many, death even became an object of morbid fascination, which for Aries, was "a sublimation ... of the erotico-macabre phantasms of the preceding period" (Aries, 1974, p. 61); in fact, the popularity of media programs about it shows that people have continued to be interested in the more grisly aspects of death.

As the main effect of the nineteenth century's rising investment in the empirical sciences as the primary source of true and reliable knowledge, however, society was rapidly becoming secularised. But there was also a significant sacrifice to be made; reaching a climax in the late nineteenth and early twentieth centuries, the disappearing expectation of an afterlife began to make the members of our advanced societies look upon death as an even more fearful occurrence. As a corollary to this increasing anxiety about it, references to personal death were becoming rarer in everyday conversation; as Aries saw it: "Death, so omnipresent in the past that it was familiar, would be effaced, would disappear. It is ... an absolutely unheard of phenomenon" (Aries, 1974, p. 85). As will be seen in Part II of this chapter, due in part to the advent of two world wars in the first half of the twentieth century, paradoxically, the increasing absence of references to personal death in everyday conversation was accompanied by an upsurge in published writing about thanatology, the scientific study of death. In fact, Aries' observation that the human preoccupation with their relationship with death had disappeared was only superficially true; although it was not discussed in everyday conversation, the subject was very much alive in the twentieth century and indeed, became one of the most challenging issues medical professionals and public intellectuals alike have ever had to confront.

Is our fear and rejection of personal death now so widespread that medicine is under pressure to keep postponing it?

For some decades now, people have been challenging human mortality. In 1967, Dr James Bedford was the first person to have himself cryonically preserved; this involves low temperature freezing of the body after clinical death has been declared, in the hope that a resurrection can take place when medical treatments not currently available have been found. Although this practice is considered unscientific, it still continues; for example, as of 2014, 250 cryonically-frozen corpses remained in cold storage in the USA. (Retrieved from https://en.wikipedia.org/wiki/Cryonics)

More contemporary and appealing purveyors of eternal life, cosmetic companies have recently been claiming that they can slow, prevent, or even reverse the ageing process. In order to appear medically credible, they often use words like 'telomeres', 'leucocytes', 'stem cell therapies' and other terms which are intended to sound scientific, and provide eye-catching illustrations of cells and chromosomes in their advertisements. According to Dr John Rasko, Professor of Medicine at the Institute of Cancer Medicine and Cell Biology at the Royal Alfred Hospital, Sydney, their claims are exceedingly far-fetched; rather than the transformative agent that the advertisements promise, their offer of unproven stem cell-based interventions is very concerning to genuine clinicians (Rasko, 2016, May 10, Radio National Breakfast). Nonetheless, the burgeoning of these advertisements suggests that, in what seems like a tacit collusion between the community and its medical scientists, increasing numbers of us think that even though all of our predecessors have succumbed to it, modern medical advances will eventually provide us with the power to hold death off indefinitely. Indeed, the wish to avoid ever having to die is for some becoming so intense that the likelihood cannot be acknowledged that, even if death could be endlessly postponed, the life being so desperately clung to would become ever more marginal, and its social cost, astronomic.

Can we learn to face death by studying its acceptance in ancient societies?

As a corrective to the present search for eternal life, Aries advocates a return to the way people accepted their mortality in primitive societies. Claiming that in those days, the common man's attitude to death was "tamed" by the social control exerted by the church over the population, Aries argues that death in primitive societies was experienced as "familiar, close and softened" (Aries, 1974, p. 2). However, sociologist and author of *The loneliness of dying*, Norbert Elias, disagrees with Aries; he criticises as over-idealistic Aries' portrayal of death in primitive societies as "tamed", pointing out that life and death in feudal and mediaeval states could be "passionate, violent ... and wild", and that people often died in great agony (Elias, 1985, pp. 12–13). According to Elias, Aries relies on preconceived opinion rather than citable evidence when he asserts that in earlier times, people died serenely and calmly, and he depends too much on romantic epics for his accounts of ancient and mediaeval life and death (Elias, p. 12). However, Elias does agree with Aries' view that in past centuries, death and dying were regarded as in the nature of things, and were spoken of far more openly and frequently than they are now (Elias, p. 15). Whether or not the members of earlier societies were truly death-accepting, the current hope that death can be neutralised would be regarded by them as the stuff of fairy tales.

Elias and Aries also agree that the socio-economic revolution of the nineteenth and twentieth centuries was a major agent of the present repugnance towards death, and of the public expectation that eventually, all ills will be curable. But for Elias, as well as being desired, the idea of living forever had first to be widely imagined as even *possible*. For this to happen, in the course of becoming civilised, society had to undergo a process which Elias identified as *internal pacification* (Elias, p. 48). That is, once societies became civilised states protected from invasion and violence through the maintenance of law and order by those who alone were authorised to bear arms, their populations were largely shielded from death and injury by sudden and violent attacks from within or without. Elias argues that it was only when people could safely block out awareness of its ever-present proximity that they could even begin to picture a life free of the constant threat of death (Elias, p. 48). Ironically, however, in continuing to ward it off, present-day society's attempts to turn a blind eye to the existence of personal death have only made its inevitable reality more alarming, and even harder to face when it can no longer be ignored. After all, treating death as too frightening to acknowledge can only add to its already intimidating reputation.

In another area of agreement, Elias and Aries both note that despite the historical gains made in quality of life and death, people in contemporary society often suffer lonely and unaccompanied deaths in institutions (Elias, p. 15). As they see it, although in the past intimate others could be violent and cruel, their being in close and constant contact could also offer a kind of comfort at the deathbed that it is impossible for modern institutions to provide. By contrast, however, as Clive Seale observed in the previous chapter, it is quite possible to die alone at home, and hospitals can at least offer the security of medical care to the dying. Further, MacArtney et al. found that, while many of the dying might express a wish to die at home, in practice, they raised very little resistance to being transferred to hospital (MacArtney et al., 2016). Perhaps institutionalised dying is not as tragic for the patient and their loved ones as Aries and Elias believe it to be; when they are dying, perhaps people's attitudes to where their best security lies may have changed in the last forty years. However, the point they make is well-taken; as many more are doing nowadays, institutions caring for the dying need to move away from maintaining a sterile, isolating hospital environment, towards the creation of settings which are more companionable, homely and family-friendly.

Is it too late to return to the natural attitudes to death found in ancient societies?

Supposing for the moment that despite Elias' criticism of it, there is some truth in Aries' view of the nature of dying in ancient societies, would it be possible for our death-avoidant contemporary society to return to the more natural and open attitude to personal death that Aries believes was characteristic of ancient societies? Observing that modern dying has been "furtively pushed out of the world of familiar things", he asks: "Is it impossible for our technological cultures ever to regain the naïve confidence in Destiny which had for so long been shown by simple men when dying?" (Aries, 1974, pp. 105–107).

There are two difficulties raised by Aries' premise that "simple men" in ancient societies approached death with "naïve confidence in Destiny". Firstly, our socio-economic circumstances have completely changed since the ancient times to which he is referring. Even if people in ancient societies did accept death in the way that Aries claims, it was not necessarily due to their supposed simplicity; rather, it was the result of their poverty and their lowly status, and of the social control that the combined forces of the feudal lords and the church were able to exert over them in all matters of life and death. Fast-forwarding to the twenty-first century, there has been a seismic shift in the way we *collectively* construe death. As sociologist Geoffrey Gorer points out in *The pornography of death*: "The natural processes of decay have become ... as disgusting as the natural processes of birth and copulation were a century ago" (Gorer, 1994, p. 74). Underlying the absence of talk of death in contemporary social life, what is unacceptable to us about death – its ugliness and its deadly power – now appears as fiction in horror stories and films (Gorer, 1994), where for example, a heroic doctor will triumph over grisly death's savage attacks on the vulnerable. Our experience of what death is like is becoming largely relegated to fiction or the national news; at the same time, the delivery of ever greater longevity – even immortality – is increasingly talked about as if it were a real possibility. Accordingly, prolonging life, and if that is not possible, micro-managing a 'good death', are much sought after; in this kind of ethos, trusting Destiny to mediate a peaceful acceptance of dying is unlikely to be a popular option.

Secondly, the development in the Middle Ages of concern about 'my death' signalled that a radical change was occurring in how people *individually* thought about their own death. Prior to this, as long as he was a chattel for the use of the feudal lord, an obedient servant of the church and in general, the object of the will of others, a serf would have had little opportunity to develop a mind of his own. His mental energies would have been devoted to sustaining the routines and functions of his small domain, and to the pragmatics of his role in relation to the overlord, the church, his family and the neighbours. Now, if I am to have an attitude to something both personal and abstract like "my (potential) death", I must first be able to represent it symbolically to myself in words or images, which I have come to know have the same meaning for me as for my community. But this could not happen; until the emergence of the idea of 'my death' in the Middle Ages, neither my concepts nor my vocabulary would have included the words to represent my individual death to myself. Since I would have been unable to think about it consciously, in common with everyone else, I would most likely have been quite satisfied to adopt the readymade judgement of the church about what my death signified, and what to do when it was imminent. Accordingly, although I would have taken it to be just how things were, my attitude to dying would have owed a great deal to how I was programmed to think and behave, and very little to my personal acceptance of death as natural.

Much as Aries may long to return to it – whether or not it was simple and accepting – this stage in the development of human consciousness has gone beyond recall.

Part II. The twentieth century: The rise of thanatology

Despite the existence of an increasing silence about matters of death and dying in everyday conversation, the twentieth century saw a surge in thanatological writings by scientists and public intellectuals. It is the purpose of this section to examine some of the significant theories in this field, and to find out what light that they can throw on the wider psychological and social aspects of death.

Understanding our attitude to death: Focus on subjective experience

Scientific research designed to understand from a psychophysical standpoint what our own death means to us, burgeoned during the twentieth century. Often engaged simultaneously in clinical activities and psychological research, investigators working within the positivist tradition of theory-building gathered quantities of individual data for studies which they hoped would yield generalisable conclusions.

An outline of five significant twentieth-century contributions follows:

- Sigmund Freud's theory of the death drive in *Beyond the Pleasure Principle* (1920)
- Herman Feifel's study of death in *The meaning of death (*1959)
- Elisabeth Kubler-Ross' Five Stages of Grief in *On death and dying* (1969)
- Ernest Becker's theory of *The denial of death* (1973)
- Norbert Elias' study of *The loneliness of the dying* (1985)

Sigmund Freud's theory of the death drive (1920)

In 1920, Freud published *Beyond the Pleasure Principle*, which, though written quite late in his career, was ground-breaking; in it he claimed that humankind has "an urge in organic life to restore an earlier state of things", or the innate potential to return to an inorganic or inanimate state (Freud, 1920, p. 308). While he did not believe that the human unconscious knew death, Freud postulated the biological existence of a death drive or instinct which, in contrast with the drive towards survival, sex, propagation and creativity, had the function "to assure that the organism shall follow its own path to death" (Freud, 1920, p. 311). Still controversial, the death drive theory was part of Freud's attempt to account for his patients' apparent compulsion to re-enact or repeat destructive and traumatic events, a clinical finding which could not be accommodated within his lifelong view that human beings' mental lives were governed by the pleasure principle. Whether or not our path toward death can properly be called a drive, Freud's claim that its directive force was innate suggested that, by an imperceptible process which can never be under our conscious control, we are from conception programmed to die.

Arguably, if anyone had until then assumed that in general, death arrives only when we have become vulnerable to disease or accident, they would have found Freud's claim that we are born already set to die confronting. Moreover, his suggestion that from the outset, as well as impulses toward good living, we all harbour instincts which draw us as if within a force field towards destructiveness and death, may to some have seemed beyond belief. But the claim that we are born with the inscription of our death already in place is probably accepted in most advanced societies by now, with the possible exception of those who believe that in due course, we may not have to die at all.

A second unsettling feature of Freud's death drive proposition was its suggestion that although we are born already programmed to die, for most of our lives we have no intuitive knowledge or awareness of it; it is beyond our awareness and control. Typically, until we are put on notice of death from a grave illness, we live each day as if our lives will never end. While for Freud, our unconscious mind has no cognisance of our own death, contemporary psychodynamic thought inclines towards the view that – just as in being born – our death is inscribed in our genetic endowment and hence, must be part of our unconscious landscape. Arguably, though, how we will respond to facing our own death is unknown to us in advance of our doing so, and is ordinarily unknowable.

Herman Feifel's study: The meaning of death (1959)

An American clinical psychologist working extensively with war veterans, Herman Feifel was not the first to pay attention to the study of death; as early as 1903, Russian microbiologist and Nobel Laureate, Elie Metchnikoff, had advocated including dying in the study of human life, but his suggestion was never taken up (*Encyclopaedia Britannica Online*. Retrieved from https://www.britannica.com/biography/Elie-Metchnikoff). Despite the traumatic slaughter of two world wars, the tendency to ignore death and dying as worthy of research continued, and by the mid-twentieth century, their prospective death was still not being discussed even with terminally-ill patients. In the 1950s, however, thanatology began at last to emerge as an interdisciplinary research interest, and Feifel's writings on personal death are generally regarded as its pioneer.

Strongly influenced by psychoanalytic theory, Feifel needed no persuasion to be convinced of Freud's view that human death is part of life from the beginning, though he was less optimistic that the general public would become convinced of it:

> If we accepted death as lodged in our bowels from the very beginning, energies not bound up in continuous strivings to shelve and subdue the idea of death could be available to us for the more positive and constructive aspects of living.
>
> (Feifel, 1990, p. 541)

Rather than diminishing us, to Feifel, understanding death represented a resource for the living: "The attitudes concerning [death], and its meaning for the individual, can serve as an important organising principle in determining how he conducts himself in life" (Feifel, 1959, p. 128). For Feifel, accepting our mortality strengthens our capacity to be honest with and accept ourselves, and recognition of limits in general is an essential component of maturity.

Although like Aries, he felt that talking about death had become taboo in everyday life, Feifel found that in the consulting room, both the well and the mentally ill people whom he interviewed wanted to be able to speak directly and honestly to their doctors about it. His first publication, *The meaning of death*, was an empirical and interpretive investigation of his main finding that death is feared. Amongst his subjects, there was a widespread apprehension about death; they feared the unknown, and dreaded the loss of their sense of identity and their most cherished relationships. Reflecting on this, he wondered if the fearful anticipation of death is "the prototype of human anxiety" (Feifel, 1959, p. xiii), a construct which was later taken up as fact by his compatriot, Ernest Becker.

There were substantial issues that were widely shared amongst his patients. Listening to their concerns, Feifel came to believe that those facing death needed a mentor to help them to review their lives, to revisit and to try to repair wasted years, undone tasks, lost opportunities and unused talents and finally, to face their remorse for "the avoidable evils which have been done" (Feifel, 1959, p. 127). However, crucial as reviewing one's life is, it is equally necessary to prepare for its ending: "The evolution of an *ars moriendi* prior to death is needed" (Feifel, 1990, p. 541). But these concerns are not just a modern phenomenon, thrown up by our secular age. According to Aries, resisting despair and instead, seeking an understanding of one's own narrative from within the intense experience of facing one's own death – "la mort de soi" – is not a new aspiration (Aries, 1974, p. 52). Rather, it has existed from time immemorial – inherent in the philosophical polemics of ancient Greece and Rome, resurgent in the Middle Ages in Europe and then, revived in Western society during the last century. But Feifel did add something of his own to this extensive body of thought; he suggested that specialist mentors for the dying were needed. Excellent as it is, however, his recommendation reveals a potential problem; in a society as death-avoidant as our own, finding people willing and qualified to fill the role of mentor would not be easy.

With a background in the positivist tradition, Feifel sought to provide quantities of data to support his thesis on behalf of the dying, but he was also interested in the details of individual cases, in how people think – including himself. His response after *The Meaning of death* was published in 1959 to a mixed reception was typically insightful. Having declared that the meaning of death was important to everyone, he explained that he had himself first developed a need to understand it while still young; having seen a dead uncle being laid out, he had had the thought that knowing that we will die could veto one's most ardent dreams. Later, he came to understand that the fear of being nullified by death's implacable existence could be overcome by love – love for friends and family, and for one's fellow man (Woo, 2003).

Open recognition of the relevance to its integrity of a researcher's personal reasons for undertaking a particular investigation is a comparatively recent development; ahead of his time, Feifel acknowledged the motives for his need to explore what death means to us more than sixty years ago.

Elisabeth Kubler-Ross' Five stages of grief in the dying (1969)

Probably best-known for her book, *On death and dying: What the dying have to teach doctors, nurses, clergy and their own families* (1969), Swiss-American psychiatrist, Elisabeth Kubler-Ross, believed that professional people involved with the dying had a responsibility to investigate what being faced with death meant to their patients. As with Feifel, her concern for her patients stimulated a wish to talk to her in those who had been told, or had intuited, that they were terminally ill. From the findings of her many interviews with patients and their families, Kubler-Ross famously distilled a hypothesis that those facing death generally pass through the following five psychological states of grief and mourning:

- i) Denial and isolation – withdrawal, becoming uncommunicative and disallowing the diagnosis, before partially accepting it
- ii) Anger at the injustice and cruelty of the diagnosis: "Why me?" – sometimes accompanied by resentment toward and envy of well people
- iii) Bargaining for more life in return for making a special contribution of some kind, usually carried out secretly
- iv) Depression: not so much reactive to the diagnosis, as preparing for the impending loss of all love objects ahead and thus, facilitating the state of acceptance

v) Acceptance – not happiness, but almost void of feelings, beyond fear and despair and needing only a quiet, comforting presence until death comes; the pain and struggle are over. It is time for "the final rest before the long journey". (Kubler-Ross, 1969, pp. 38–137)

There have been a number of forceful criticisms of Kubler-Ross' hypothesis; some of these have been presented by Stroebe, Schut and Boerner in a 2017 paper entitled: "Cautioning health-care professionals: Bereaved persons are misguided through the stages of grief". A number of these critics have taken her paradigm to be "progressivist", or prescriptive of how we should die, when in fact, whatever her followers or readers have made of her work, she herself explicitly rejected this description: "These [coping mechanisms] … will last for different periods of time and will replace one another or exist sometimes side by side. The one thing that usually persists through all these stages is hope" (Kubler-Ross, 1969, p. 138). Her description of the 'acceptance stage' has also been criticised as creating a persecuting ideal which must be achieved if we are to experience a 'good death'. But according to Kubler-Ross' description of it, acceptance is not an achievement; it is the reverse, a state of letting go, spontaneously activated within the dying individual as death approaches, and beyond the domain of conscious striving. Rather than the result of an effort of will, or an effect of religious belief or of reasoning, for those participants in this study who experienced acceptance it seemed to be a state of being, an attitude activated within them as they readied themselves for the approach of death. Arguably, criticisms which imply that Kubler-Ross' hypotheses are meant to be taken as dogma rather than as guidelines to be used flexibly as a resource, may be doing her intentions an injustice.

Another group of critics argues that to accept the "five stage labelling" might not only control a dying person's behaviour, but the very meaning of the experience itself. A typical proponent of this view, William Gavin, argues that: "Stories, as opposed to stages, may or may not be progressive in nature; they may well proceed in zigzag fashion and may contain contradictions" (Gavin, 1995, pp. 141–142). Moreover, binaries like "denial versus acceptance" do not take account of people's shifting and ambivalent mental states, or their wish to rebel against their fate or their management; with research into dying, the narrative should be allowed free rein and be as "thickened up" as possible (Gavin, 1995, p. 142). In fact, Kubler-Ross kept verbatim tape-recorded case notes on her interviews with the dying and their families, but she would have had to iron out individual differences and inconsistencies in this originally "thick" data in order to produce summaries suitable for her hypothesis-building; this procedure is inherent in the nature of the cross-sectional, quantitative form of data analysis with which she worked. By contrast, Gavin's criteria for retrieving valid data would perhaps be more suited to a longitudinal, qualitative analysis with a smaller group of subjects. Nonetheless, his charge that Kubler-Ross put her studies into question by reducing real warts-and-all people to statistical ciphers is serious; it suggests that her conclusions cannot be trusted, because they were based on entities that were so categorised and oversimplified that they may no longer have represented the individuals from whose data they were drawn. In effect, Gavin is arguing that because there is such a disconnect between Kubler-Ross' "Five stages" hypothesis, and the patient interview data on which it was supposedly based, the validity of her conclusions is rendered dubious.

There will often be a tension between the need to produce streamlined summaries and classes based on individual data for quantitative statistical use toward theory building, and the need to use a qualitative approach in order to retain and build in rich personal details; for this reason, a mixed methods approach is being adopted by some contemporary researchers. Arguably, given that Kubler-Ross' work was based on detailed interviews with patients and their families, she would have been better served if she had first used qualitative methods to carry out an exploratory study of her rich data, and based on its findings, had only then initiated a mixed methods or purely quantitative investigation with theory building in mind.

A further criticism of Kubler-Ross' work relates to the assumptions underlying the collection and interpretation of her data. Like Feifel, Kubler-Ross subscribed to psychoanalytic theory but unlike him, she used it as a virtual template to frame what people in our society think personal death is:

> It is inconceivable for our unconscious to imagine an actual ending of our own life here on earth, and if [it] ... has to end, the ending is always attributed to a malicious intervention from the outside by someone else .... In our unconscious mind we can only be killed; it is inconceivable to die of a natural cause or of old age. Therefore, death in itself is associated with a bad act ... something that ... calls for retribution and punishment.
>
> (Kubler-Ross, 1969, p. 2)

According to Kubler-Ross, these "bad acts" of ours are a universal source of guilt and shame; for example, if we hate someone or wish them ill, we feel responsible if they suffer or leave us, because: "We cannot in our unconscious mind distinguish between a wish and a deed" (Kubler-Ross, 1969, p. 3). In short, Kubler-Ross believed that our fear of death is an artefact of our expectation of being killed as a punishment for an actual or imagined "bad act", and that moreover, if we fail to grasp this fundamental truth, we will never be able to understand "the otherwise unintelligible communications of our patients" (Kubler-Ross, 1969, p. 3).

It is not within the scope of this investigation to discuss the merits and demerits of Kubler-Ross' psychoanalytically-based assertions themselves. What does need to be considered, however, is how far taking such a position *a priori* would have influenced her approach to interviews with patients, and coloured her interpretation of their data. Seen through the theoretical filter that people fear death because they feel that it is a punishment for wrongdoing,

Kubler-Ross would tend to elicit from her participants responses of a punishment-fearing kind, such as angry defiance, guilt and shame.

It is not obvious from its content what part her psychoanalytic bias might have played in the evolution of Kubler-Ross' "Five stages" theory. Arguably, however, in a field still as full of unknowns as the experience of dying, preconceptions of any kind would have been best kept critically in mind or if possible, avoided, in case the outcome of the research seemed more like a manifesto – as some of Kubler-Ross' critics have implied that it was – than the result of a rigorous investigation. That is not to say that "The five stages of grief" hypothesis is vacuous, but it does suggest that further work would be needed in order to clarify under what circumstances and to whom, Kubler-Ross' findings might apply. In the present study, where no one was in denial, four out of the five participants asked "Why me?" although in contrast with Kubler-Ross' subjects, their responses covered a wide range from self-blame to well-considered, thoughtful answers, and only one complained of feeling punished – unjustly, as it happens, and therefore, pleading not guilty. On the other hand, decisions about whether or not to do deals in the hope of obtaining more time in return for suffering brutal treatment were indeed made by all the participants, and finally, to the accompaniment of sad farewells, four out of five of them did arrive at the stage of acceptance. Overall, then, while there are important differences between them, there is also some congruence between the Kubler-Ross' findings and those of the present study.

In a later book, *Death: The final stage of growth* (1975), further experience had apparently mellowed Kubler-Ross' views: "Death does not have to be a catastrophic, destructive thing; indeed, it can be viewed as one of the most constructive, positive, and creative elements of culture and life" (Kubler-Ross, 1975, p. 2). And whatever the final truth value of her "Five stages" hypothesis, her way of thinking about the experience of dying radically changed the practice of end of life care, and was central to the development of the hospice and palliative care movements. Devoted to the psychiatric profession and to her patients, perhaps at heart, Kubler-Ross preferred hitting the campaign trail with an *ars moriendi* package for all, to the meticulous calculation and weighing up of evidence in the laboratory.

Ernest Becker's theory: The denial of death (1973)

Cultural anthropologist Ernest Becker's Pulitzer Prize-winning book, *The denial of death*, was published in the year before he died; it was a work which combined the philosophies of Kierkegaard and Norman Brown and, like Feifel and Kubler-Ross, the dynamic psychology of psychoanalysis. Taking up an idea first mooted by Feifel, Becker claimed that all human anxiety does indeed originate in the fear of death – indeed, that if we were unable to remain at all times distanced from this fear, we could not remain sane. Typically, therefore, by deploying psychological defences, we repress or deny the fear of death throughout life. As Becker pointed out, although we are physical human beings, we also exist as symbolic entities in a symbolic world of meaning. On this premise, he reasoned that by living as far as possible through our symbolic selves, we are capable of suppressing the paradox of our mortality that, although intent upon surviving, we know that we must die. Note that where this investigation seeks to discover a *resolution* of the paradox, Becker's belief that man can never afford to face it at any level precludes this possibility.

Accordingly, Becker contended that our narcissism allows us to *transcend* our dilemma by symbolically re-creating ourselves in our imaginations as heroic and invincible in our ambitions in life, and in our standing in the world. To justify himself as an object of primary value: "[Man] must stand out, be a hero, show that he *counts* more than anything or anyone else" (Becker, p. 4). In Becker's view, we are able to do this by using our cultural values and religious beliefs to provide us with the raw material we need to embody our heroic illusions; in this way: "the complex symbol of death is … transcended by man [through] a belief in immortality" (Becker, p. 24). However, Becker warns that there is a cost to our maintaining this delusional system; immortality projects are prime motivators of human conflict such as wars, religious bigotry, genocide, and racism. Even worse, there is a risk of diminishing returns or even of the collapse of the system, as our societies become more secular and their belief systems less noble, rendering religious and other heroic themes less available to us. In short, according to Becker, as far as facing death is concerned, man is damned if he does and equally, damned if he does not.

Though common enough, denial of personal death is not as universal a condition as Becker claimed; for example, no participants in the present study demonstrate it. Perhaps Becker's attention was focused on our public face, on the absence of discussions about our feelings about personal death in everyday social life, but perhaps, to own our feelings about death, we need to be in a secure and private context. Further, given that Becker's theory is as monothematic and lacking in empirical underpinning as it is, it is doubtful that it could do all the heavy lifting required of it by the claim that although the fear of death is fundamental to all human anxiety, it can be surmounted by mass quasi-megalomaniac delusions. Further, as Ryan and Deci argue, it must be asked if people's search for significance and meaning within the values of their own culture can be reduced to a set of defensive processes designed to ward off the fear of death (Ryan & Deci, 2004). In that case, surely all such quests would by now have been extinguished through a lack of genuine substance. Finally, although Becker refers to the importance of developmental processes in human maturation, his account does suggest that their potency is generally a function of repressive defences rather than its being the other way around, a position unlikely to be corroborated by developmental psychology.

From a different perspective, a number of recent papers question the idea that the "denial" of personal death regularly said to exist in medical contexts is always true denial – that is, that a patient's knowledge of the approach of death in the foreseeable future has been repressed from consciousness. Rather, several papers show that being "in denial" about personal death is not the all-pervading circumstance that Becker took it to be; being "in denial" about one's death is by no means universal, and it is also challenging to diagnose. Indeed, physician Tara Tucker claims that the routine misdiagnosis and dismissal of the reticent dying as being 'in denial' is in effect professionally negligent (Tucker, 2009, p. 1108). Social psychologist Camilla Zimmermann argues that it is becoming accepted in modern society that failure to communicate about one's approaching death can be construed as being 'in denial' and accordingly, seen as an obstacle to a 'good death' (Zimmermann, 2007, p. 297); she suggests that such a view might lead to pressure being put on reticent patients to speak up, or be considered uncooperative with treatment. On a similar theme, Gavin declares that far from denying one's death, turning away may represent the individual's aggrieved protest about having to die (Gavin, 1995, p. 191). Finally, according to sociologist Alan Kellehear, we have never been a death-denying people, and in any case, there is no transglobal proof that fear of death is universal (Kellehear, 2007, pp. 56–58).

Although Becker's theory is no longer widely accepted, it continues to form the basis for the research and theoretical development in Terror Management Theory by USA social psychologists Jeff Greenberg, Sheldon Solomon, Tom Pyszczynski and others.

Norbert Elias' study: The loneliness of the dying (1985)

In 1985, eight years before his death aged ninety-three, sociologist Norbert Elias first published *The loneliness of the dying*, a work which discusses trends in the management of the dying which are still relevant in contemporary society. By now himself a member of the ageing cohort in modern European society, Elias writes in a style which combines professional objectivity with fraternal compassion. As with the research in my own study, Elias' treatise is based on the premise that the experience of facing death is group-specific and as such, varies greatly between societies – it seems a natural process, but much of it is learnt (Elias, 1985, p. 5). His work begins with the prelude to death, old age; he claims that the aged have become the object of all that the young want to deny in themselves – the repugnance and embarrassment about certain physical functions, and the relative loss of control and independence in old age. Most disowned of all, however, is the proximity of approaching death: "which both as a process and a memory image, is one of the great bio-social dangers in human life ... now banished ... away from public social life" (Elias, p. 12). But of course, increased life expectancy does not alter the fact that in the end, we do still die (Elias, p. 77).

According to Elias, we conceal the facts relating to death – our dead are removed swiftly, odourlessly, hygienically and behind the scenes – and exclude it all from normal life (Elias, p. 29). As life in our society becomes longer, death further postponed, and the sight of the dead and dying rarer, death can effectively be forgotten for most of our lives (Elias, p. 7). In relation to how we see life, Elias argues that our present society is characterised by a high degree and specific pattern of individualisation, in which people see themselves as fundamentally independent beings who feel that it is right to further their own interests without including anyone else (Elias, p. 34). But there is a certain aridity involved in living like this; even if someone is satisfied that their life was fulfilling, and their dying is understood to be necessary, personal death is often experienced as lacking in reason or meaning (Elias, p. 62). According to Elias, this is the direct legacy of our high level of individualistic living; for him, there can be no meaning in a person's life or death that is independent of what that life means to other people (Elias, p. 55). He has a warning for us about continuing to live in this way; when confronted with the dying of someone we know, lacking a sense of empathic connection, we are liable to feel embarrassed and inadequate, and to have nothing to say to them (Elias, p. 24).

In past times, old and dying people usually remained within the living area of the family and the neighbours, and whether treated kindly or brutally, they were not left alone (Elias, pp. 72–75). By contrast, Elias finds that the modern institutions which accommodate our elders and dying are often regimen-focused, devoid of feeling, and lacking personnel with any affective bonds to the dying, all of which increases their isolation; its ultimate form must be to die as many do, in the terminal ward or ICU. Although he is aware that we cannot render all ordinary deaths accompanied, calm and peaceful, Elias makes a plea; it would certainly be much better if the dying did not have to feel an embarrassment to or a burden on friends and family. Death is the end of the person, but there is solace for them in knowing at the last that they will live on in people's memories. Indeed, according to Elias, we need to recognise that the real pain of death for everyone is that, whatever we may have imagined to be the case in life, we have always been part of each other (Elias, p. 66).

Repression and concealment of the finitude of human life is not a peculiarity of the twentieth century; although people have long resisted it, they have also tried to understand why they must die. While literally dying alone is preferred by some people, there is a certain sense in which we must all die alone; since we cannot share the little world known only to ourselves which will die with us, it cannot be otherwise. And while there are culturally-based images of death which, at both the individual and the collective level, can be terrifying – the Grim Reaper depicted in television advertisements, for example – Elias does not think that death itself is terrible; it is simply our natural end: "One passes into dreaming and the world vanishes, if all goes well"

(Elias, p. 66). For Elias, the real loneliness of the dying lies in the failure in our society to recognise, and to move to redress, the deep pain that is caused by the experience of being left alone to die by those to whom we are attached.

The loneliness of the dying is a reflective, introspective study by a veteran sociologist rather than an empirical account focused on factually-based claims and statistical comparisons. Elias is concerned about the isolation which he thinks has become characteristic of our individualistic society in both life and death; having emerged in the Middle Ages and granting as it did the status of human beings to many who had once been mere chattels, individualisation was once a sign of social progress. For Elias, however, our individualism has become so extreme that it cuts us off from each other; in his view, there is no meaning in a person's life or death that is independent of its meaning to other people. He distinguishes the essential loneliness of the dying – a consequence of our inability to share the little world known only to ourselves – from the inhumane loneliness of dying in the absence of friends and family, perhaps in a clinical setting with no one to whom we are attached being there for us. For Elias, the first of these is simply a necessary fact of nature, but the second is a tragedy, both for the one who must die like that, and for those who allow it.

Since Elias recorded these sorrowful reflections, however, lonely dying like this may be starting to become less common; death notices in the papers regularly announce that the person who has died was "surrounded by" his or her family. Perhaps this is more than just a change in how we treat our dying; the prominence given in these public announcements to the attendance of the family suggests that we are becoming aware that our presence at a loved one's death is profoundly meaningful, to us and to them.

Testing Elias' claims against the present investigation

Did the participants in this study experience either the inner world isolation or the loneliness due to the social rejection and neglect of the dying described by Elias? All five participants wrote about the essential solitude when facing death of living in one's own inner world which, although it occurs on various occasions throughout life, is inseparable from the experience of dying and perhaps, reaches its purest form there. Rather than a turning away from others, for them, the inner world experience was somewhere private to go when respite was needed from the constant hum of the life around them. In fact, all participants in the study had close relationships with spouses and other family members, as well as with friends and colleagues. Dying slowly of cancer, they all had the time and capacity to weave hospital care and family presence together; none seem to have experienced the cut-off and extended, lonely dying in an institution which so troubled Elias and indeed, although they all grieved profoundly over losing their loved ones forever, none of them expressed any persistent fear of being left to die alone.

Accordingly, the findings in this investigation do not support Elias' concern that there is a generalised and increasing tendency to deny that we are part of each other and hence, that people are being left to die cut-off and alone. However, it is impossible to know whether or not the circumstances of this particular group of articulate and well-supported participants is typical of trends in the population in general.

Part III. Philosophical opinion on death, ancient and modern: Does death cause us harm?

Given the distress it often causes us to think about it, philosophers have for two millennia debated the question of whether or not humanity's fear of death is justified. One of the earliest formulations of an argument that the fear is not justified was put forward by Greek philosopher Epicurus, and further developed by Roman poet and philosopher, Titus Lucretius Carus. Ever since then, philosophers have continued to debate Lucretius' argument, and although none of them has succeeded in defeating it, the way that the grounds of the debate have changed is informative. In particular, the argument put forward in answer to Lucretius by contemporary American philosopher, Thomas Nagel, demonstrates how differently death is viewed now in comparison with its portrayal in ancient times.

Two theories about death from ancient Greece and Rome: Epicurus and Lucretius

In the fifth century BC, some centuries prior to the advent of the debate about whether or not death does us harm, Greek philosopher, Plato, declared that as the body and the far wiser soul were ultimately separate entities, the soul could only be liberated by the death of the body:

> It has been proven to us by experience that if we would have pure knowledge of anything we must be quit of the body – the soul herself must behold things in themselves: then we shall attain the wisdom which we desire … not while we live, but after death; for while in the company of the body, the soul cannot have pure knowledge.
>
> (as cited in San Filippo, 2006, p. 5)

Accordingly, in order to ensure the immortality of the dead through their remembrance by the living, funerals in Plato's day were meticulously-observed formal rites, and mourning rituals continued for some time afterwards. Belief in life after death was widespread; ancient Egyptian, Greek, Roman and American Indian burial sites all displayed the dead surrounded by artefacts for use in the afterlife (San Filippo, 2006, p. 5).

By the first century BC, on the other hand, the fear of death seemed to have taken precedence over the expectation of an enlightened afterlife, and the philosophical advice given to the populace had become less reflective, and more instructive. The earliest recorded proponent of this approach was Greek philosopher, Epicurus, the author of the first existence argument:

> When we exist, death is not yet present, and when death is present, then we do not exist. So death is nothing to us
>
> (as cited in Lei, 2007, p. 1).

But as Lei points out, Epicurus' argument that death need not be feared is completely objective; it makes no reference to a subject, a person, who may be fearful of or harmed by their awareness of death's hegemony (Lei, 2007, p. 1). On the other hand, in the first symmetry argument on record, Epicurus' follower, Roman poet and philosopher, Lucretius, does recognise the existence of a subject:

> Life is granted to no one for permanent ownership, to all on lease. Look back now and consider how the bygone ages of eternity that elapsed before our birth were nothing to us. Here, then, is a mirror in which nature shows us the time to come after our death .... Does it not appear more peaceful than the deepest sleep?
>
> (Titus Lucretius Carus, 50 BC/2001, Book 3, s. 971–976)

As Lei observes, the basis of Lucretius' symmetry argument that one need not fear death is that post-mortem non-existence is not fearful because it is relevantly similar to pre-natal non-existence, and no one has ever claimed that pre-natal non-existence is fearful (Lei, 2007, p. 1). According to Lei, in setting out to show that death does no harm by refuting the subject's anticipatory fear of the state of being dead, Lucretius provides an additional dimension for Epicurus' existence argument. However, Lucretius' argument would not be effective against the fear of death *per se* or of dying, which have since the Middle Ages been the main causes of man's death anxiety. As eighteenth-century philosopher and scientist, Francis Bacon, declared: "I do not believe, that any man fears to be dead, but only the stroke of death" (Bacon, 1765, p. 574). In the time of Lucretius, philosophers had no knowledge of the conceptual frameworks needed to address a widespread anticipatory fear of '*my* death', or of dying. As was noted in Part I of this chapter, if the concept of '*my* death' existed at all, it was probably confined to the educated and aristocratic classes throughout feudal times, and did not become widespread until the mid-Middle Ages; perhaps Lucretius was ahead of his time in addressing individuals at all.

But a revolutionary change was on the way. Once the populace as a whole had individuated, and in doing so, had developed self-consciousness and the ability for reflexive awareness of their thoughts and feelings, a new universe of communication was opened up. From then on, philosophers, playwrights, poets and indeed, all creative thinkers could speak from their inner worlds to and about the inner worlds of their respondents. It was from this by now long-established, once new world that twentieth century American philosopher, Thomas Nagel, addressed Lucretius, the scholar from ancient Rome.

Thomas Nagel's reply to Lucretius

In reply to Lucretius' argument, Nagel focuses on the premise which asserts that pre-natal non-existence is symmetrical with post-mortem non-existence. He raises two linked objections to this statement. Firstly, he does not agree that death's non-existence is simply the mirror image of pre-natal non-existence and therefore, he claims that it is reasonable to regard them differently. Having previously argued that the experience of life is of value *per se*, he claims that any loss of expected life causes the individual harm: "Any death entails the loss of *some* life that its victim would have led had he not died at that earlier point" (Nagel, 1979, p. 7, his emphasis). Secondly, he takes up the matter of pre-natal non-existence: "The time prior to a man's birth is time in which he would have lived if he had been born not then but earlier" (Nagel, 1979, p. 7); adroitly, though without supporting his claim, Nagel argues that if he had been born earlier, the man would simply have been someone else. In conclusion, he argues contra Lucretius' view that death deprives us of nothing, that in fact, it is death's deprivation of the good of life, rather than the prospect of eternal non-existence, which arouses our fear of it. In my own experience, however, this argument is only true where the fear of death as non-existence has been tested and put aside, while the love of life remains intact.

Nagel's argument against Lucretius turns on two assumed values which in fact, Lucretius did not share with him. The first of these is Nagel's attribution to each of us, a state of passionate ownership regarding '*my* life' and '*my* death', whereas in referring to '*our* death', Lucretius is thinking of death as an objective, generalised phenomenon, terminating a lifespan which we have never owned, but have merely occupied temporarily as tenants. Secondly, Nagel claims that '*my* death' deprives us of the greatest of all values, the goods of life, to which we are deeply attached and for him, it is the prospect of this loss which is the main cause for our fear of death. Lucretius does not mention this at all. Given that the notion of the anguish of '*my* death' and the associated losses of *temporalia* had not emerged as universal concerns until the Middle Ages, Lucretius and Nagel were not even sharing a hymn book, let alone singing from the same page.

Although he believes it to be so, Nagel does finally acknowledge that he has no conclusive explanation of the asymmetry that he has identified between past and future non-existence. However, he claims that:

> The sense of subjective possibility does not project itself into the past with the same imaginative reality with which it faces the future. Death is the negation of something the possibility of whose negation seems not to exist in advance.
>
> (Nagel, 1986, p. 229)

Noting here that there is an incongruity between the subjective view of personal death – the concern about '*my* death' – and the objective view of death as simply exemplifying natural law, Nagel observes that he is also well aware that his death, "like any other, is an event in the objective order" (Nagel, 1986, p. 229). When it is thought of in this impersonal way – in fact, in the way in which Lucretius regarded it – he finds it natural to feel a sense of detachment, to regard his death without too much concern, "as part of the general cycle of biological renewal" (Nagel, 1986, p. 229).

Accordingly, Nagel wonders if it might be possible for contemporary individuals accustomed to incline only toward the subjective to identify as well with the objective view, and in closing the gap between the two standpoints, to regard death with more equanimity. Ultimately, however, he sees no way of eliminating the radical clash between the two standpoints – objective and subjective – in relation to death: "We cannot rise above death by occupying [an objective] ... vantage point that death will destroy" (Nagel, 1986, p. 231). Unlike Lucretius, Nagel therefore concludes that our problem with contemplating our own death has no prospect of objective resolution; indeed, he declares that "to recognise that is to come as near as we can to living in the light of the truth" (Nagel, 1986, p. 231).

Elias' comment on Nagel: A psycho-social approach to facing personal death

As Elias sees it, the mainstay of Nagel's position is that death is a problem for human beings because they know beforehand that despite their most assiduous precautions, they could die at any time; "It is not actually death but the knowledge of it that creates problems for human beings" (Elias, 1985, p. 5). For some, like Nagel, and especially in the face of a terminal diagnosis, this may stimulate an attempt to come to terms with it. According to Elias, it is the anticipatory image of death in the consciousness of the living, not the anticipation of death itself that arouses fear – for example, in modern society, of a car smash, or being ravaged by cancer; he does not regard fear of death as an innate predisposition in human beings, as Nagel assumes. Accordingly, Elias suggests that a remedy for the members of a particular society's fears of death might lie in re-educating public attitudes towards a more benign characterisation of death.

Further, Elias claims that at present, there is another, even more insoluble problem associated with how we regard death; since we have no way of preventing it, we have to repress our fear of dying alone, and as more and more of us do so, a vicious cycle is becoming established. Since for Elias, it is the build-up of collective psychological patterns of unconscious beliefs about dying that is the active ingredient in our fear of it, death's supposed cosmic loneliness is a fundamental aspect of that. As observed in Part II of this chapter, Elias' own belief is that death is not terrible; it is our natural end.

Participants in the present study illustrate both the insights represented in Nagel's portrayal of the vacillations between the subjective and the objective views of death, and Elias' view that particular images of how one might die may be the key to what frightens us about it. Ultimately, however, the fears and nightmare visions simply fall away; as four of the participants discovered, acceptance of death is possible, and as Elias observed, and one participant at least exemplified, it can even deliver a last phase spent not in terror, but in a kind of dreamy and gentle, drifting away into oblivion.

Summary of chapter

Part I of the chapter introduces the concept of death as being as much a social construct as a biological event; as it is used in this study, the expression 'my death' refers to our understanding of what the experience of death is like. Then follows an account of changes in our attitudes to death over the last two millennia, from antiquity to the twentieth century; the evolution of the notion of 'my death' in the Middle Ages is central to understanding our present attitudes to death. Part II focuses on the upsurge in thinking and writing about personal death in the twentieth century. In Part III, a debate between philosophers, ancient and modern, about whether or not death causes us harm, ends the chapter.

Next follows Chapter 4, *Learning from the dying*. For those who wish to know more about the technical aspects of the study, an account is given of its research design – that is, of how the data was collected – the selection of its participants, and the methods used to analyse and present the data.

References

Aries, P. (1974). *Western attitudes toward death from the Middle Ages to the present*. P. Ranum (Trans.). Baltimore: John Hopkins University Press.

Bacon, F. (1765). An essay on death. *The works of Francis Bacon* (Vol. 1). London: A. Millar, in the Strand.

Becker, E. (1973). *The denial of death*. New York, NY: Free Press.

Elias, N. (1985). *The loneliness of the dying*. E. Jephcott (Trans.). Oxford: Basil Blackwell Ltd.

Feifel, H. (1959). *The meaning of death*. London and New York: McGraw Hill Book Company.

Filippo, D. S., National Louis University, Illinois. (2006). *Historical perspectives on attitudes concerning death and dying*. [Faculty Publications Paper 29]. Orlando, FL: Kimball Publishing. Retrieved from http://digitalcommons.nl.edu/faculty_publications/29

Freud, S. (1920/1987 version). *On Metapsychology: Beyond the pleasure principle*. Harmondsworth, Middlesex: Penguin Books.

Gavin, W. J. (1995). *Cuttin' the body loose: Historical, biological, and personal approaches to death and dying*. Philadelphia: Temple University Press.

Gilleard, C. (2002). Aging and old age in mediaeval society and the transition of modernity. *Journal of Aging and Identity, 7*(1), 25–41. doi: 10.1023/A.1014358415896

Gorer, G. (1994). The pornography of death. In J. B. Williamson & E. S. Schneiderman (Eds.), *Death: Current perspectives* (4th ed., pp. 73–77). Palo Alto, CA: Mayfield Publishing Company.

Grayling, A. C. (2016, September 3). *On the modern mind* [Interview with Geraldine Doogue, Radio National Saturday Extra]. Retrieved from https://radio.abc.net.au/

Kellehear, A. (2007). *A social history of dying*. Cambridge: Cambridge University Press.

Kubler-Ross, E. (1969). *Death and dying*. New York: Macmillan Publishing Company.Kubler-Ross, E. (1975). *Death: The final stage of growth*. Englewood Cliffs, NJ: Prentice-Hall.

Lei, K. (2007). *Defending Lucretius' symmetry argument against the fear of death*. (Master's thesis, Georgia State University). Retrieved from https://scholarworks.gsu.edu/cgi/viewcontent.cgi?article=1018&context=philosophy_theses

Lucretius: Titus Lucretius Carus. (50 BC/trans. M. F. Smith, 2001). *De rerum natura: On the nature of things* (Book 3, s. 971–976). Indianapolis, IN: Hackett Publishing Company.

MacArtney, J., Broom, A., Kirby, E., Good., P., Wootton, J., & Adams, J. (2016). Locating care at the end of life: Burden, vulnerability, and the practical accomplishment of dying. *Sociology of Health and Illness, 38*(3), 479–492. doi: 10.1111/1467-9566.12375

Nagel, T. (1979). Death. In T. Nagel (Ed.). *Mortal questions* (pp. 2–10). Cambridge: Cambridge University Press.

Nagel, T. (1986). Birth, death and the meaning of life. In *The view from nowhere* (pp. 208–232). Oxford: Oxford University Press.

Parker, M. (2011, November 25). Body or soul: Why we don't talk about death and dying. *The Conversation*. Retrieved from https://the conversation.com/body-or-soul-why-we-dont-talk-about-death-and-dying-4354

Rasko, J. (2016, May 10). *The pseudoscience of anti-ageing* [Interview with Fran Kelly, Radio National Breakfast]. Retrieved from http://www.abc.net.au/radionational/programs/breakfast/the-pseudoscience-of-ageing/7400358

Ryan, R. M., & Deci, E. L. (2004). Avoiding death or engaging life as accounts of meaning and culture. Comment on Pyszczynski et al. *Psychological Bulletin, 130*(3), 473–477. doi: 10.1037/0033–2909.130.3.473

Stroebe, Schut, & Boerner. (2017). Cautioning Health-Care Professionals: Bereaved persons are misguided through the stages of grief. *Omega, May 75*(1). doi: 10.1177/0030222817701499.PMID: 28395639

Tucker, T. (2009). The culture of death denial: Relevant or rhetoric in medical education? *Journal of Palliative Medicine, 12*(12), 1105–1108. doi: 10.1089/jpm.2009.0234

Walter, T. (1991). Modern death: Taboo or not taboo? *Sociology, 25*(2), 293–310. doi: 10.1177/0038038591025002009

Zimmermann, C. (2007). Death denial: Obstacle or instrument for palliative care? An analysis of clinical literature. *Sociology of Health and Illness, 29*(2), 297–314. doi: 10.1111/j.1467–9566.2007.00495.x

4 Learning from the dying

Introduction: Why a study of the experience of our dying elders is needed

As this is a study of what it is like to die in a more or less ordinary and timely manner, the five memoirists who were chosen as research participants, and who have provided us with such invaluable data about their experience of dying, were all in their sixties and seventies. The book is not about the more uncommon deaths – from homicide, suicide, accident, the effects of war or any other catastrophe – nor is it about the deaths of the young; these are often traumatic deaths, and require studies of their own.

Given that dying is inevitable, it may surprise the reader to learn that, as far as I am aware, this small qualitative study represents the first systematic research into how, from the initial diagnosis on, a group of terminally ill older people prepared themselves to die. Not only that, it is also the first study in which the data to be analysed are composed entirely of what the dying people themselves have to say. While many accounts of the reflections of the dying have been published, they are generally anecdotal, illustrative of particular themes within a larger overall narrative, rather than presented in entirety, and in their own right.

Death studies researchers Clarke, Korotchenko and Bundon (2012) found that, even though the elderly dying in our society often face a slow, heavily medicalised death – sometimes over years – from a combination of morbidities and chronic conditions, there had been little investigation of older adults' attitudes towards death, or of their experience of the dying body (Clarke et al., p. 1399). As Hugh Willmott (2000) observed in Chapter 2, contemporary sociological literature had at that point made no reference to the experience of dying. Finally, when in 2019, I turned to the Internet to discover what was on offer there under the heading of 'Preparing for death', I found that the books and articles listed there were either offering advice on the management of dying loved ones, or advertising educational books and public events about how to manage ageing and becoming more frail. They were all produced or organised by the living, for the living. Not one was an account of their experience, written or described, by the dying.

DOI: 10.4324/9781003392088-4

Given the depth of the silence on the matter, it was likely to be challenging to find enough memoirs written by dying people themselves to furnish the data for the inquiry. I began with a search on the Internet, but this process supplied only a few suitable texts. Literary reviews and news items also provided some appropriate titles, but the majority were suggested by colleagues, friends and family members with academic interests, who knew of my research interest. In all, only twenty-four memoirs finally came my way, but as the research is the first of its kind, a modest beginning is appropriate; the study is exploratory, rather than theory-building. Further research may develop the many themes and trends which even this small study has revealed.

To preface the discussion of its research design, a recapitulation is needed of the 'burning questions' investigated in the study:

1 *What is it like to face death?*
2 *If our most basic instinct is to survive, how can we become ready to relinquish life and accept death?*

The chapter is divided into two parts:

Part I. Designing the research
Part II. Introducing the participants

Part I. Designing the research

For those to whom such methodological detail is vital to their assessment of a study's value, this chapter provides some detail of how the memoirs were analysed, and conclusions drawn about what it is like to face death. Further, the chapter identifies what the data can tell us, and what it cannot. For example, it may be expected that the study would focus on the participants as *persons*, and that the psychodynamic analysis of their writings about facing death would therefore be, in effect, psychoanalyses of their personalities. But this is not the case. The objects of the study are in fact the participants' *attitudes to death and dying*, and it is these *attitudes* that are the subject of psychodynamic analysis, ultimately supplying most of the data.

The research design and tools required for the collection and organisation of data from the study participants' memoirs are identified in what follows. A summary of the overall design of the collection and presentation of the study data is provided, followed by a detailed account of the procedures used in the analysis and organisation of the data.

First, the summary: To allow us to learn how their attitudes to impending death evolved over time, the experiential narratives written by the five participants have been analysed using qualitative content analysis. An inductive procedure, this allows the researcher to examine the collected data item by item, and to develop categories and themes from an initially undifferentiated mass of information.

Once the relevant items in the memoirs have been extracted, identified and organised into coherent groups, the discussion of their meaning and significance is presented in two different formats.

a) an across-participant, chronologically-based data analysis and its discussion is presented in the next three chapters, as follows: Chapter 5, *Reacting to the news*: *Diagnosis,* Chapter 6, *Living with dying,* and finally, Chapter 7, *Acceptance.*
b) in order to use the same material to identify challenges in contemporary end of life care, the data groups are first reorganised into thirty-two themes, and then, further refined to form eleven clusters of related themes. In Chapter 8, *Themes in the experience of dying*, the items in these data clusters are discussed in relation to the wider literature on care of the dying, and recommendations made for its improvement.

Secondly, to ensure transparency and comprehensiveness in the reporting of how the data was gathered and analysed, a more detailed account of the research procedures used in the study is provided. The two discrete but interdependent formats involved are:

i) The choice of qualitative research for the study
ii) The research paradigms selected for the study

The choice of qualitative research for the study

Since it is suitable for studies which focus on the language and meaning of the participants' accounts of their experiences and perspectives facing death, qualitative research has been employed in this study (Sullivan, 2010). As the preferred alternative to the quantitative approach to research – which investigates and reports on large-scale trends – qualitative research permits an examination in depth and in detail of the dying experience of a few people. Accordingly, the data was collected through a close reading, re-reading and analysis of the participants' memoirs, all of which were written by their own choice, and within their own natural setting. Qualitative research specialists, Miles, Huberman and Saldana (2014), advise that relatively little standardised instrumentation is required for data collection in this kind of investigation; rather than making use of impersonal questionnaires, the researcher brings to the investigation "deep attentiveness and empathic understanding" as essentially, its main instrument (Miles et al., p. 9).

There are many different approaches to qualitative research, but they have in common an interest in using the data to explore "meaning-making", rather than statistical differences or relationships (Gibson & Riley, 2010, p. 60). As Miles et al. observe, given that it examines the use of words by a writer and their interpretation by the reader, qualitative research is bound to contain a relatively higher level of subjectivity in terms of the meaning attributed to the words used by each party. Arguably, however, as in this case the native language of researcher and memoirists is the same, there would be a sufficient area of shared understanding involved in plain language interchanges for the use of words as data to achieve a satisfactory degree of reliability and validity.

Once assembled, the memoirist's words and phrases can be broken into segments, and coding which denotes categories of meaning – such as the memoirist's reaction to the initial diagnosis – can be applied to all passages chosen for their relevance to the study objectives. Ultimately, the researcher can go on to construct data sets and sub-sets, clusters and themes from the coded data; it will then be the main task of the study to use the data "to describe the ways people in particular settings come to understand, account for, take action and otherwise manage their day-to-day situation" (Miles et al., p. 9). For theoretical reasons, where a relevant body of literature exists, interpretations that must be made in the process of constructing the data sets and themes may be chosen as the most compelling possibility to hand. On the other hand, where no such literature exists – as is the case with this pioneering study – the choice may be made on grounds of credibility and trustworthiness.

Given that they are based predominantly on words, "Qualitative data are not so much about behaviour as they are about *actions* (which carry with them intentions and meanings and lead to consequences)" (Miles et al., p. 11, their emphasis). Accordingly, researchers need to be aware that if strongly motivated to do so, participants can use words to gear their responses to how they would like to be seen. It follows that every researcher needs to be alert to statements which do not quite add up, or seem to strike a wrong note. Further, participants will also be affected by the specific social context which they occupy – in this case, for example, two of the participants had strong religious affiliations – and this may influence how their words are interpreted by a non-affiliated researcher. In order to remain as free as possible of personal bias, then, it is essential that the researcher seeks to maintain a non-judgemental stance at all times.

To an impartial observer, the '*local groundedness*' of the data is actually a potential strength, because "the influences of the local context are not stripped away but are taken into account. The possibility for understanding latent, underlying or non-obvious issues is strong" (Miles et al., p. 11, their emphasis). As they observe, such data is rich and holistic, providing 'thick', or substantial descriptions of a participant's experience which can have the ring of truth, and as readers will find out from reading Chapters 5–7, they can strongly impact the reader. Further, given that it is usually taken flexibly and over time, qualitative data can tell us what is really going on in some vital aspect of the subject's life or as here, in their experience of dying. As well as its creativity in generating hypotheses, with its emphasis on people's lived experiences, qualitative data is well suited to "locating the *meanings* people place on the events, processes and structures of their lives and for connecting these meanings to the *social world* around them" (p. 11, their emphases). In sum, it is ideally suited to a small-scale study of dying.

The qualitative research paradigms used in the study

For this study, I have used two different qualitative data paradigms in order to maximise what the data can yield: case study, and autothanatography, a paradigm developed from ethnography.

Case study

This paradigm provides a framework for the selection and exploration of the memoirs written by the five research subjects selected for the study. Given that the cases are the participants' attitudes, this multiple-respondent case study is intended to deliver more varied and compelling evidence in answer to the research questions than a single-respondent case study could do. Moreover, according to social scientist Robert Yin (2014), case study is the preferred method when, as here, the study is contemporary, the researcher has little or no control over behavioural events, and the main research questions are 'how' or 'why' some particular social phenomenon works in the way that it does.

Doyen of case study proponents, Robert Stake (1994), further refines the criteria for its application: "Case study is not a methodological choice but a choice of object to be studied" (p. 236); as stated in the introduction to this chapter, the cases are the participants' attitudes to their own dying and death. Further, according to Stake (2000): "As a form of research, case study is defined by interest in individual cases, not by the methods of inquiry used" (Stake, 2000, p. 435). It allows a researcher to carry more than one case study on simultaneously, with each one being itself a concentrated inquiry. Pointing out the rewards of studying "the ordinary and the everyday", Stake (2000) makes it clear that the use of a qualitative research paradigm is not *faute de mieux*, or the result of a lack of appropriate quantitative approaches. Rather, as he sees it, "Opportunity to learn is of primary importance ... Isn't it better to learn a lot from an atypical case than a little from a seemingly typical one?" (pp. 446–447). In accordance with this view, the present study examines each case of participant attitudes to their own death in depth, and in detail. Occurring as it does in an untrodden field, this investigation sets out neither to draw formal generalisations of its own, nor to add to any other pre-existing theory or body of knowledge; it is a pioneering, and hence, exploratory study.

With the introduction of the participants and their struggles with terminal illness now imminent, we are about to see how powerful an experience of getting to know each person case studies can offer; it is as if we are there *with* them, identifying with their struggles, rather than being kept at a distance, and told *about* them. Readers are provided with a vibrant and true-to-life account of the participants' often harrowing, but at times, uplifting experiences. Thus, the reader will have the opportunity to fully understand the characters and the events of each case, and to draw their own conclusions about the nature and quality of the study as a whole.

Stake (2000) offers us some typically pithy guidance on the ethics of carrying out valid case study research: "Place your best intellect in the thick of what is going on", and remember that the work is observational, interpretive and above all, reflective (p. 445). Regarding the researcher's ethical responsibilities, his advice is trenchant: "Qualitative researchers are guests in the private spaces of the world. Their manners should be good and their code of ethics strict" (p. 447).

Autothanatography

In general terms, autothanatography is a longitudinal, qualitative research instrument which, in this case, employs document analysis to provide data for the case studies. Evolved from autoethnography and ultimately, the paradigm of ethnography, it is a form of autobiographical life writing which deals with the period of the writer's final illness and death. As a discourse drawn from the writer's own life experience, it focuses on personal memories, and on self-observational and self-reflective data; accordingly, there is an emphasis on introspection, and on both interpersonal- and self-analysis (Chang, 2008). The knowledge acquired through the use of this paradigm draws on the rich and subtle meanings of people's lives, and is largely experiential rather than conceptual.

Autothanatography has unusual, and sometimes challenging features. Reflecting on the impossibility of testifying to our own deaths because death annihilates the first-person witness, Linnell Secomb (2002) observes that the nearest approximation must be to write about near-death experience, or about "being-towards-death" (p. 33). For her, if death is immanent in life, survival is not an escape from death, it is its internalisation; if this is right, both death- and survival-seeking would represent fundamental inscriptions in our instinctual endowment, and knowledge of death as our final destination must be carried within us throughout life. Thus, when we face impending death, our task is not so much to construct a challenging new scenario, as to undo or bypass the repression which, as Freud claimed, has until that point prevented us from accessing what we have always known. As a driving force for the writing of autothanatography, then, 'survival and death' are for Secomb not so much irreconcilable opposites, as different ways of looking at death while still in life.

E. S. Burt (2009) sees autothanatography as a type of confessional text. He argues that those who read our memoirs post-mortem can, in so doing, retrieve a sense of the otherness that represents us in death – an otherness which, though we can never know it ourselves, can nonetheless become accessible to someone else. According to Burt (2009), autothanatography therefore "has the potential to witness for alterity unrecoverable by the subject ... the writing of the death of the subject" (p. 6). As I experienced and described it in Chapter 1, death is often experienced as the Great Other or the Great Unknown, a kind of negation of ourselves as the positive entity;

grappling with its death, however, as was explored in Chapter 2, the "I" can never hope to determine that alterity, or conceptualise its own death. Nonetheless, there are those who engage in a monumental struggle to do so; this book gives an account of six such individuals – the five participants, and myself. And the saga of our struggle to identify the Great Other of death is addressed to you, the reader.

Death is ineffable; yet we strive to understand what it means to us even if in the end, we may not be able to find the words to describe it. Dying, on the other hand, can be experienced and described.

As this most demanding of projects required, all of the authors in the study were accomplished writers, and accustomed to being open and articulate about their thoughts and feelings. Moreover, since their aim in writing was to reflect upon and record their final experience of life, they wanted to communicate with themselves and their audience as honestly and clear-sightedly as possible. That is not to say that bias can be completely excluded; for example, a writer might on occasion overstate his or her position for fear of failing to reach an audience that they know they will never play to again. Certainly, all of the participants wanted their memoir to represent an authentic account of their experience of living and dying, but this did not imply that everything they wrote was meant to be verifiably accurate. What they wanted was a chance to chronicle as authentically as possible their subjective experience of dying of cancer.

How far their contributions can be thought of as representative of the experience of the dying might also be queried. After all, they represent a highly specific group; it may not be possible to take accounts given in autothanatographies by such sophisticated thinkers as typical of the experience of the terminally-ill population in general. On the other hand, where attitudes expressed in the data analysis are found to be shared by most or all members of the participant group, or strike the reader intuitively as common to us all, it would suggest that they may also occur in the wider population.

In fact, in terms of honesty and spontaneity, autothanatography may be a more trustworthy text than its more mainstream relative, autobiography. Comparing the two, Kelly (2009) claims that, although traditional literary theories endorse autobiography as presenting a unified, coherent sense of self, grounded in a humanist empirical tradition which assumes that the author had access firstly, to a privileged source of their own life's meaning, and secondly, to a past self with a high degree of unity and consistency, the idea that autobiography possesses such an authoritative quality may well be illusory. Kelly argues that by contrast, autothanatography is more true-to-life, because it embraces "more open-ended elements" like mutability, change and transience, which are actively involved in the writer's coming to terms with death (p. 33). Life writer, Suzanne Egan (2001), observes that, even though autothanatographers' body-selves lack an imaginative future, their repeated efforts to name their experience becomes "a moment-to-moment wrestling match with the angel of death", and despite the struggle being unwinnable, with amazing frequency, it results in "the naming of the self", the revelation of their identity (Egan, 2001, para. 6). Indeed, according to Richard Momeyer, in choosing how to confront death, "we choose our very character" (as cited in Egan, para. 6).

In fact, autothanatography is actually more direct and immediate, more grippingly 'alive' than autobiography, because it never becomes a retrospectively polished history; it is often written on the run, right up to the final, heart-stopping, finishing-line. On this view, in the present study, the need for accurate reporting benefits from the likelihood that autothanatography has more in common with the spontaneity of live interviews than does the more premeditated, refined form of autobiography. Moreover, given that the writers may not be alive for long after publication, they might reasonably be supposed to be less concerned with projecting an image into the future, and more with communicating immediate thoughts and feelings. For the participants in the present study, a sense of the urgency of their mission to tell the world about the experience of having to leave it is never far away.

Footnote: My role as 'Insider researcher'.

Given that I shared the experience of facing death with my participants, my research is to that extent an example of 'insider research'. Now, while my role as researcher did not affect what my participants wrote, the possibility exists that my experience of facing death myself could have distorted my interpretation of what they had to say about their experience. For example, Rooney observes that as an insider researcher, one might unjustifiably assume commonalities between oneself and one's subjects because of having shared their experience; if sufficiently distorting, a bias of this kind could even invalidate the study (Rooney, 2005, Conclusions). On the other hand, inside knowledge can alert one to pertinent issues in the participants' material, and allow one to reflect on them in a more accepting and informed way. For Rooney, while these questions are important to raise, they are difficult to resolve, and in any case, given that they apply to some extent in all research, they will always necessitate constant monitoring (Rooney, 2005, Conclusions). In fact, the possibility of my slipping into joining the participants as a notional group member does not arise in the case of the dying as typically, dying is done alone. Indeed, two of the participants referred to the loneliness of dying. However, I did notice a potential problem with contamination in one domain; early on, when a participant I was studying finally stopped writing and died, I felt grief. Accordingly, having seen how deeply involved with each individual I could become, I always allowed myself enough time to process and close each substantial interaction with any one participant, before undertaking the analysis of the next.

Part II. Introducing the participants

Following the application of my selection criteria to the original group of 24 memoirists, six persons remained involved in the study – myself, and five memoirists; these five writers make up the group referred to in Chapters 5–8 as "the participants".

The participant group

Jenny Diski, Philip Gould, Christopher Hitchens, Michael Mayne and Cory Taylor

As a group, the participants were educated and literate, able to produce an autothanatography which was richly individual and expressive. They all faced their condition squarely; at no time did any of them react to their diagnosis with denial. As persons, they were all reflective, articulate and self-aware, and strongly motivated to make their last book as honest and full of meaning as possible. In particular, they wanted to examine and share their thoughts about the meaning of their life and death, and since none of them could know how long they would be alive to do so, there was an immediacy in their writing, a forward movement towards the end that they all knew awaited them. All active members of accepted groups in society, they were not recluses, eccentrics or loners; of distinct personalities, they also came from widely different social, economic and family backgrounds.

As yet, perhaps only the articulate and expressive write autothanatographies, but it seems also to be the case that committing oneself to writing about what the experience is like mobilises a profound and sustained interest in the life that is coming to a close. As a form of life writing, it may become increasingly popular.

A short biography of each participant

Jenny Diski. (2016). *In gratitude*. London and New York: Bloomsbury Publishing.

Jenny Diski, FRSL. Writer.

Born: 8th July, 1947, London.

Died: Lung cancer, 28th April, 2016, aged 68, Cambridge.

Father: James Simmonds, rag trader, confidence man. Deserted the family when Diski was 6, died 1966.

Mother: Rachel Rayner, estranged from Diski in the 60s, died sometime in the 1980s.

Sponsor: Doris Lessing, novelist, died 2013, aged 94.

First husband: Roger Diski, ethical travel pioneer. Married 1976, separated 1981 and later divorced.
Daughter: Chloe Diski, married, two infant children.
Second husband: Dr Ian Patterson (known as 'The Poet'), Director of Studies in English, Queens College, Cambridge. Married 2008, until Diski's death in 2016.

Jenny Diski was the only child of Jewish East End working-class/semi-criminal, immigrant parents. Diagnosed at sixty-six with an inoperable tumour of the lung during a routine check-up on her pulmonary fibrosis, she wrote her memoir initially as a monthly column for *The London Review of Books*; she wanted to give an account of her thoughts about her life, her cancer treatment, and facing death. In fact, she spent much of the memoir examining and trying to resolve a conflict which had haunted her since her teenage years. As a child, she was the object of conjoint sexual abuse masquerading as 'play' by her parents and when, as an adolescent and at their invitation, she spent four years living with Doris Lessing and her teenage son, Peter, the dynamic configuration of being 'played with' by a powerful couple was reactivated, entrapping her afresh. She had no awareness of this unconscious traumatic pattern as the source of her reactions to her conflicts with the Lessings, or in her wrist-cutting, drug-taking destructiveness towards herself when young. Until her death, she was tormented by an ultimately futile preoccupation with what she experienced as being unjustly held responsible for the failure of the Lessings' experiment in fostering her.

Finding a way to personal fulfilment through writing, she was a prolific and successful writer of both fiction and non-fiction; she was prepared to write about disturbing and difficult topics, and her material was always well-researched and deftly handled. Indeed, equipping herself with the best information available became her way of maintaining her equilibrium in all aspects of her life.

Her first marriage to Roger Diski in 1976 ended after five years, but they remained close friends until, in 2011, Roger accidentally drowned while swimming off the coast of Sierra Leone. During her last sixteen years with her second husband, academic Ian Patterson, to whom she refers as 'The Poet', she finally gained both intellectual companionship and warm support; she was also able to enjoy a loving relationship with her daughter, Chloe, by Roger Diski, and her two grandchildren.

Under the pressure of troubled thoughts about her life and her fear of a terrifying death by suffocation, she ended her memoir abruptly, with some indications of a breakdown in her capacity to think coherently; she died some weeks later.

Philip Gould. (2013). *When I die: Lessons from the death zone.* Great Britain: Abacus.
Lord Philip Gould, Baron Gould of Brookwood, M. Sc. (LSE). Political consultant to New Labour, UK.

Born: 30th March, 1950, Woking.
Died: Oesophageal cancer, 6th November, 2011, aged 61, London.
Wife: Dame Gail Rebuck, The Baroness Rebuck of Bloomsbury, Chair: Penguin Random House Publishers, London. Labour member, House of Lords.
Adult daughters: Georgia, M.A. Leader (Labour), Camden Council, London. Grace, B.A. Early stage investor consultant.

Philip Gould was the younger child of British parents, both of whom were dedicated teachers. Handicapped by dyslexia, he was no scholar when young, but eventually, he became a successful advertising executive who went on to take a Master's degree in the history of political thought and eventually, to be a political consultant to the British New Labour Party. When first diagnosed with non-metastasised oesophageal cancer at fifty-eight and given a fifty percent chance of survival, he responded with typical optimism. However, despite his having kept the cancer at bay for two years with chemotherapy and two strenuous rounds of surgery, his condition again deteriorated and in 2011, some three months before his death, he received a terminal diagnosis. While the cancer ended his life, Gould never believed that it had defeated him.

Always a workaholic, Gould felt guilty about neglecting his beloved family, and when first diagnosed, about having let them down by overworking and neglecting his health. He was not much given to inner conflict – indeed, he was invincible in getting his own way – but as his death approached, he was confronted by his wife, Gail, with repeatedly setting her home-making projects aside, and moving the family on to suit his work requirements. Sincerely remorseful, he apologised, and was forgiven; always a loyal couple, he and Gail were able, with his two daughters, to meet his death as a close and united family.

Gould believed that we all have the power within ourselves to transcend death by cancer, and to emerge stronger for it. First published in *The Times*, his memoir was intended to convey this message to the world: If you accept death, and look it in the eye, the fear of it disappears. As he approached death in an at times ecstatic, quasi-mystical state of mind, he declared that although living in the 'Death Zone' was inevitably sad at times, accepting one's oncoming death while living life to the full could also be transformative, and a time of intense happiness.

Christopher Hitchens. (2012). *Mortality*. New York & Boston: Twelve Books.
Christopher Eric Hitchens, PPE (Oxon). Writer, lecturer and public intellectual.
Born: 13th April, 1949, Portsmouth, England.
Died: Oesophageal cancer, 15th December, 2011, aged 62, Houston, Texas.
Father: Eric Hitchens, Commander, British Royal Navy.
Mother: Yvonne Hickman, Jewish. Parents separated; mother died by suicide in 1973.
Brother: Peter, born 1951, Christian, socially conservative journalist.

First wife: Eleni Meleagrou, Greek Cypriot, one son, one daughter. Married 1981, divorced 1989.
Second wife: Carol Blue Hitchens, American writer. Married 1991, one daughter.

Christopher Hitchens was the elder son of middle-class British parents; his mother was Jewish, and in adulthood, Hitchens adopted her Jewish identity. His parents' marriage broke down and as a young man, Hitchens had to identify his mother's body following her suicide. A well-known journalist and public intellectual who loved debate and spirited company, Hitchens was a campaigning left-wing socialist who lived life in the fast lane. As a lecturer and polemicist, he was well-known for his sharp-edged aphorisms and his brutal iconoclasm towards major public figures, including Princess Diana, Ronald Reagan and Mother Teresa. At sixty-one, just when he was promoting his memoirs, *Hitch-22*, he was diagnosed with stage four metastasising oesophageal cancer. He described his final memoir, *Mortality,* as being about what it was like to live while dying.

Having voluntarily undergone waterboarding in order to mount an informed criticism on its use by the US government, he had written in *Vanity Fair* that he had felt then that he was really drowning; in hospital with the cancer, he developed an anxiety about water-using procedures. Sensitive to the distorting effects of chemotherapy on his mind, he also came to fear that he might become unable to distinguish his cancer treatment and palliative care from torture and execution. Accordingly, his memoir was intended to publicise the need for vigilance regarding hospital procedures. Originally published as instalments in *Vanity Fair*, the book features a first chapter devoted to a trenchant denunciation of Christianity and its followers; Hitchens wanted it to be on record that no one should believe the rumours that he expected his pious opponents would circulate that he had recanted his antitheism on his deathbed.

To express his understanding of why we all have to die, the final entry in his memoir – recorded just before he died – quotes a passage in Alan Lightman's 1993 novella, *Einstein's Dreams*, in which Lightman explains that immortality would be disastrous for the human race. He imagines that if no one ever died, we would all be burdened with oversight by an infinite list of fathers and mothers, their fathers and mothers, and so on, ad infinitum, forever unable to become free and independent spirits. For Hitchens, freedom of thought and speech was precious enough to be worth the price he had to pay for it.

Michael Mayne. (2006). *The enduring melody*. London: Darton, Longman & Todd.
The Very Reverend Michael Clement Otway Mayne, KCVO. Dean Emeritus of Westminster. (Mayne had been knighted, but clergy do not use titles.)
Born: 10th September, 1929, Harleston, Northants.
Died: Cancer of jaw, 22nd October, 2006, aged 77, Salisbury, Wilts.

Father: Reverend Michael Ashton Otway Mayne, died 1933, by suicide.
Mother: Sylvia Ellis, had two further marriages and was twice widowed.
Wife: Alison McKie, married 1965.
Children: Sarah, community nurse, married with children.
Mark, secondary school principal, married with children.

Michael Mayne was the only son of British parents; his clergyman father had suicided by throwing himself from the church tower, leaving no note. Mayne had no memory of his father and, left alone with his bereaved mother, he felt overwhelmed at times by her turning to him when she felt unhappy and in need of love.

While studying at Cambridge he enjoyed acting, but finally decided to train as a priest. Thereafter, he served in various parishes and roles until invited to become Dean of Westminster; he fulfilled this role competently and independently, allowing such morally controversial figures as Oscar Wilde, Edward Lear and A. E. Housman to be commemorated in the Abbey. Warm and empathic, with his wife Alison, he created a close and loving family and a loyal group of friends.

In 2005, at 76, he was diagnosed with non-metastasised cancer of the jaw and began the first of two rounds of harrowing treatment. For Mayne, writing about his ordeal offered two rewards – firstly, an opportunity to test his beliefs, the "enduring melody" of his life – and secondly, a chance to share his experience as a comfort to others. His "enduring melody" had three strands: first, the belief that human love and relationships indicate that God's love for us is infinite: secondly, that God exists in the beauty and order of the natural world and thirdly, that there are transcendent experiences in which we can discern God and his creation. Actually, Mayne acknowledged some difficulty in feeling God's presence and at times, experienced him as remote. Referring to his father's suicide and his betrayal of himself and his mother, Mayne recalled his fatherless childhood as lonely and cold. In the intense atmosphere of the struggle to survive, he seemed to become aware that there was a link between God's elusiveness for him, and his lost father. In time, he was able to resolve the two conflicts together – to extend forbearance to his father, and to realise that for him, God's loving presence was mediated through the care of his friends and certain health professionals.

In early May 2006, Mayne was finally cleared of cancer and hesitantly, he terminated his memoir and prepared to return to everyday life. However, not long afterwards – as he reported it in an addendum to the memoir – the cancer reappeared, and was terminal. He also revealed that his few treatment options at that stage were unpleasant and unpromising; he and his wife intended to refuse them, preferring quality to quantity in whatever time remained to him. He died a few weeks later.

Cory Taylor. (2016). *Dying: A memoir.* Melbourne, Australia: Text Publishing.
Cory Taylor. B.A. Screenwriter and author.

Born: 1955, Southport, Queensland.
Died: Melanoma-related cancer, 5th July, 2016, aged 61, Windsor, Queensland.
Father: Leslie, airline pilot, later unemployed.
Mother: Everil, teacher. Parents divorced when Taylor was young.
Older Siblings: Sarah and Eliot
Husband: Shin Koyama, Japanese-Australian artist. Married 1983.
Adult sons: Nat and Dan.

Cory Taylor was the youngest of three children of peripatetic parents who, when she was a small girl, lived in far-flung places like Kenya and Fiji because of her father's employment as an airline pilot. Her two older siblings were in Australia at boarding school, and she spent more time in her adored mother's company than with other children. With the parents' acrimonious marriage breakdown and the subsequent estrangement of her father from the family, Taylor continued to be her mother's close companion until she left home. In her twenties, while living in Japan, she met her husband, artist Shin Koyama, and began a family life that was divided between Brisbane and Japan; she had a fondness for both, but never felt fully at home in either.

Diagnosed in 2005 with a terminal melanoma behind her right knee, Taylor survived for more than ten years. For some time, she seems to have been relatively free of gravely debilitating symptoms, but was left helpless following a seizure from brain cancer several years after being first diagnosed. Surgical intervention postponed her death for long enough to allow her to write her final book, *Dying: A memoir*. Prior to the cancer diagnosis, Taylor had been a successful screenwriter and author of children's books; once facing death, however, she decided to fulfil a long-held plan to write adult fiction. Her first novel was the prize-winning *Me and Mr Booker* (2011), and another well-reviewed novel, *My beautiful enemy*, followed in 2013. Having become acutely aware of the silence surrounding death, from June to August, 2016, she also participated in several ABC programs about what it was like to be dying; these included the ABC's "You can't ask that", in which she answered viewers' no-holds-barred questions about it.

Throughout her life, Taylor remained close to her beloved mother, but by the time she had developed cancer, her mother was in a nursing home with dementia. Recalling her mother introducing her to euthanasia and to the Exit International movement, Taylor believed retrospectively that her mother had wanted Taylor to help her to end her life; she felt that she had failed her mother because she had not done so. Perhaps afraid that she might suffer similarly if she were to experience a total loss of control, Taylor joined Exit International and acquired a euthanasia drug for use if needed. In the end, however, she did not take it; she died in a hospice in 2016.

Summary of chapter

The processes followed in the collation of the participants' data and the procedures used in its analysis, have been described in this chapter. In all, the memoirs yielded seven main and nineteen sub-sets of data, the analysis of which is to be carried out in an across-participants format. When required by the complexity of the participants' contributions, the discussion will need to include some detailed psychological analyses of the data on their attitudes to death and dying.

I wish to acknowledge the gift of the participants' intimate reflections, and to state that I feel privileged to have worked with them.

The complete narrative will be presented in the next three linked chapters, as follows:

Chapter 5, Reacting to the news: Diagnosis, Chapter 6, Living with dying, and Chapter 7, Acceptance.

References

Burt, E. S. (2009). *Regard for the other: Autothanatography in Rousseau, DeQuincey, Baudelaire and Wilde*. New York, NY: Fordham University Press.

Chang, H. (2008). *Autoethnography as method*. Walnut Creek, CA: Left Coast Press.

Clarke, L. H., Korotchenko, A., & Bundon, A. (2012). 'The calendar is just about up': Older adults with multiple chronic conditions reflect on death and dying. *Ageing and Society, 32*(8), 1399–1417. Retrieved from https://www.ncbi.nlm.nih.gov/pubmed/24976657

Diski, J. (2016). *In gratitude*. London and New York: Bloomsbury Publishing

Egan, S. (2001). *The life and times of Autothanatography* [Workshop Discussion Paper]. Retrieved from Pain and Suffering Interdisciplinary Research Network website: http://www.english.ubc.ca/PROJECTS/PAIN/DEGAN/HTM

Gibson, S., & Riley, S. (2010). Approaches to data collection in qualitative research. In M. Forrester & C. Sullivan, (Eds.), *Doing qualitative research in psychology: A practical guide* (pp. 99–120). Thousand Oaks, CA: Sage.

Gould, P. (2013). *When I die: Lessons from the death zone*. London: Abacus, Little, Brown Book Group.

Hitchens, C. E. (2012). *Mortality*. New York, Boston, MA: Twelve Books.

Kelly, D. (2009). Looking at death in the 'I': Rosa Montero's La function Delta as autothanatography. *The Journal of Romance Studies*, 9(1), 31–45. doi. 10.3167/jrs.2009.090104

Mayne, M. C. O. (2006). *The enduring melody*. London: Darton, Longman & Todd.

Miles, M. B., Huberman, M., & Saldana, J. (2014). *Qualitative data analysis: A methods sourcebook* (3rd ed.). Los Angeles and London: Sage Publications.

Rooney, P. (2005, May). *Researching from the inside - does it compromise validity? - A discussion.* Retrieved from Dublin Institute of Technology, Educational sciences website: http://arrow.tudublin.ie/ltcart/5/

Secomb, L. (2002). Autothanatography. *Mortality,* 7(1), 33–46. doi: 10.1080/13576270120102535

Stake, R. E. (1994). Case studies. In N. K. Denzin, & Y. S. Lincoln (Eds.), *Handbook of qualitative research* (pp. 236–247). London and New Delhi: Sage Publications.

Stake, R. E. (2000). Case studies. In N. K. Denzin, & Y. S. Lincoln (Eds.), *Handbook of qualitative research* (2nd ed., pp. 435–454). Thousand Oaks, CA: Sage Publications Inc.

Sullivan, C. (2010). Theory and method in qualitative psychology. In M. Forrester & C. Sullivan (Eds.), *Doing qualitative research in psychology: A practical guide* (pp. 17–34). Thousand Oaks, CA: Sage.

Taylor, C. (2016). *Dying: A memoir.* Melbourne: Text Publishing.

Willmott, H. (2000). Death. So what? Sociology, sequestration and emancipation. *The Sociological Review, 48*(4), 649–665. Retrieved from https://onlinelibrary.wiley.com/doi/abs/10.1111/1467-954X.00237

Yin, R. K. (2014). *Case study research: Design and methods* (5th ed.). Los Angeles and London: Sage Publications.

Preface to Chapters 5–7

A note on the presentation of the memoirists' contributions

The next three chapters present the across-participants' analysis of the memoirists' accounts of what it is like to have to face preparing to die. Three participants – Diski, Gould and Mayne – remained well enough to write complete memoirs which began with their response to the initial diagnosis, and ended in their final days or weeks of life. Hitchens also wrote an account of his experience of dying from diagnosis to death, but became so ill that despite his stoicism and determination to continue, he had to resort to jottings in the latter part of his memoir. In contrast, like Diski, Gould and Mayne, Taylor was also able to produce a complete memoir; however, having been terminally ill for ten years before she spent the final year of her life writing it, she did not cover the initial diagnosis and the main period of her experience in the same detail as they had done.

There is a further variation amongst the memoirists; while the publishers for Diski and Mayne were prepared to give the author free and unlimited permission to quote from their memoirs, the publishers for Gould, Hitchens and Taylor were not. Accordingly, I have paraphrased their contributions in a way that resembles the original tone and content as closely as possible.

Finally, there are some items in the narrative to which, as a participant-researcher who has shared the dying experience, I contribute some 'snippets' of my own.

5 Reacting to the news

Diagnosis

Introduction

While most people respond to unexpectedly receiving a terminal diagnosis with shock and anxiety, their initial distress typically gives way to a myriad of questions about what the diagnosis involves – questions like how much longer they can reasonably expect to live, how the cancer will be treated and with what hope of prolonging life, and how they can find the resources to cope with suddenly being handed a death sentence. To investigate these matters, the chapter examines, under three headings, the commonalities and the differences amongst the participants in this first phase of the dying experience. Parts II and III of the analysis of the participants' initial responses are divided into a number of sub-sections.

Part I. Why the participant wrote the memoir
Part II. Reaction to initial diagnosis (*Why has this illness happened to me? Response to symptomatic warnings; Emotional responses; How long do I have?*)
Part III. Cancer as part of the self (*Is the cancer seen as part of the self? Does accepting cancer as part of the self lead to a 'better' death?*)

Part I. Why the participant wrote the memoir

Often presented early and restated at intervals in every memoir, their reasons for writing it were of the first importance to all participants. Accordingly, in order to introduce the participants and their contributions, the narrative begins with this item.

Jenny Diski

Having just received a diagnosis of terminal lung cancer, Diski initially rejects the idea of contributing yet another cancer diary to an already overcrowded market, but soon concedes that it is inevitable: "I'm a writer. I've got cancer .... Writing is what I do and now cancer is what I do, too" (Diski, 2016, p. 11).

DOI: 10.4324/9781003392088-5

She is precise about the nature of her work: "I'm not attempting... my own autobiography: I'm writing a memoir .... It contains what I imagine and what I remember being told. Absolute veracity is not what I'm after" (Diski, p. 187). From its beginnings, *The London Review of Books* published her memoir as a monthly column and many months later, near her death, Diski expresses some satisfaction about having written it: "In... practical ways, I've done it right. I thought of these monthly essays straight away .... [T]hey give me some writing and thinking to do" (Diski, p. 211).

Philip Gould

First published in *The Times*, Gould's memoir began as a series of articles about his experience of living with oesophageal cancer. Having already experienced some of the vicissitudes of treatment, he declares that he wants everyone to know that, no matter how alarming and confronting a cancer diagnosis is, they all have the inner resources to emerge a different and stronger person. As his column had been well-received and widely-read, he had come to believe that his articles were bringing about change, and that therefore, he should continue telling his story to the end. But his determination to question cancer's power to challenge and terrify was severely tested when, after two years of at times brutal treatment, he received a terminal diagnosis, and was given three months to live. Never one to withdraw in the face of a challenge, however, Gould responds to this blow by deciding that, in order to reprogram the public's attitudes to it, he will devote the latter part of his memoir to sharing his experience of confronting death. He warns us, however, that he must first clear up a basic misconception in the way personal death is understood and communicated to the public. Only then can he try to transform the way people perceive and respond to becoming aware that they must die. Unlike the other participants, he does not identify a self-affirming or therapeutic value for himself in his memoir-writing; arguably, though, his project of rescuing people from the fear of death by cancer would have given him the same kind of satisfaction that he had enjoyed when planning the campaign to convert the British public to Tony Blair's New Labour.

Michael Mayne

On being diagnosed with cancer of the jaw, Mayne intuitively understands that everything in his *Weltanschauung* is about to change. Wanting to make constructive use of the difficult time he knows awaits him, he decides to write a memoir about his experience, which he intends to weave together with some reflections on his Christian beliefs that is already in process. "This would prove an unwanted but important test of the integrity of what I most deeply believed, both as a human being and a priest ... 'the enduring melody' of my life" (Mayne, 2006, p. xv), and: "I felt the need to write about it as honestly as [possible] ... both as a form of therapy and (hopefully) to bring something creative and redemptive out of an inevitably dark time" (Mayne, p. xv). He also hopes that, if frank and sincere, his narrative might offer comfort to other people in distress: "Sharing a common human experience ... can make the journey less lonely and help authenticate perfectly normal, valid feelings ... when we walk in the shadowlands of illness, pain or grief" (Mayne, p. xvi).

Christopher Hitchens

It is not clear what motivated Hitchens to write a memoir about dying. His memoir actually begins with a chapter on one of his most persistent adversarial targets, Christianity; the high priority he has given to stating his antitheist case had been precipitated by rumours recently circulated by his religious opponents that, as a result of having become terminally ill, he had recanted his atheism on his deathbed. To be accused of not having the courage of his convictions when cornered and worse, of being prepared to bleat for mercy, had incensed Hitchens. Accordingly, it was of the first importance to him to proclaim that, even if in some kind of half-crazed final delirium, he called for a priest, the creature so humiliating itself should not be thought of as the real Christopher Hitchens.

Cory Taylor

It has been ten years since Taylor's original diagnosis of terminal melanoma; following recent surgery for metastases in the brain and now, facing her final year of life, she has decided to write a memoir about her oncoming death. Her reasons for doing so are two-fold – firstly, to create an outline of her dying, so that both she and others can see clearly what the experience is like for her, and secondly, because writing about it has helped to make dying bearable for her. Because her attention is concentrated on telling the reader something with special significance to her before she goes, she is finding that, although her body is hurtling towards destruction, recording her thoughts keeps her attention focused on the life she still has left to live. However, it is not clear what she means by wanting to tell the reader about 'something with special significance', and she does not make it explicit. Whatever it is, perhaps it is related to her uniqueness amongst the participants in recording confidences in her memoir that she is keeping from her family. For example, she refers to protecting her husband and two adult sons from becoming aware of her long-time feelings of depression and in particular, from knowing that she has bought a drug online with which she can terminate her life, if the loss of control and dignity becomes too much for her to bear. As well as these secrets, this "significant something" may be code for a message from Taylor to her family that she is hoping that, when they first read that she has shared confidences with her memoir that she has not told them, they will be able to understand what she was going through, and why she did not want to burden them with it at the time.

Given that one may not be around when it is read, writing a memoir is always likely to be hazardous in what it reveals – especially, perhaps, a memoir about one's dying.

There are no reasons common to all the participants for writing their memoirs, but four of them emphasise the benefits of writing it *per se*, some shared, and some individually held. For Diski, Hitchens, Mayne and Taylor, focusing on the writing is beneficial as a bulwark against becoming unduly immersed in the illness, while for Gould, Hitchens, Mayne and Taylor, it is fitting, when one's life is ending, to recognise and record one's most valued beliefs and experiences. Diski and Taylor also use their memoirs extensively to retrieve and analyse significant life events and relationships, while Mayne hopes that the writing will be redemptive of a dark time. Gould is the only participant to assign no intrinsic value for himself in writing the memoir; for him, it seems primarily to be a means to launch his manifesto about how to nurture the spirit to survive cancer's ravages.

For the three male participants, the memoirs represent in part a kind of mission statement. For Gould, the objective is to set himself up as a role model for, and to bring hope and dignity to cancer sufferers and to the dying, while Hitchens' aim is to provide a ready-made rebuttal of any emergent deathbed conversion rumours and also, to share his personal experience of hospital treatment of the dying with the public. Mayne hopes that his memoir will test the resilience of his beliefs under the pressure of grave, and finally, terminal illness, and at the same time, when published, provide validation and comfort to people enduring the loneliness of suffering. As will be seen, by contrast, for the two women, sharing their reflections and some long-held regrets about personal and relationship issues with their readers is what matters; for Taylor, this process turns out to be healing, but Diski remains painfully conflicted.

No generalisations about gender predilections can be drawn from such a small sample but clearly, people confronting terminal illness do not react in uniform fashion; some may want to pursue ways to benefit humanity, while others may need to ponder unresolved personal issues, a task for which, for some, professional assistance may be of benefit. But there is one belief about which the participants were united: it is essential to resist becoming submerged in the illness, and to preserve the freedom of mind to reflect on the life that is coming to an end.

Part II. Reaction to initial diagnosis (*Why has this illness happened to me? Response to symptomatic warnings; Emotional responses; How long do I have?*)

All participants recognise that death is a natural part of the life cycle; according to Gould, it is in the natural way of things that children outlive their parents; to Mayne: "In these past weeks I have been pondering on the ordered rhythm of the seasons .... the annual pattern of death and new life" (Mayne, p. 251); to Diski: "The loss of the future children and grandchildren is unbearable, although ... quite in the way of things" (Diski, p. 239), and for Taylor, death is simply a law of nature. While Hitchens does not contribute at this point, he has more to say about human mortality in his last words before dying. Referring to the final observation in Alan Lightman's 1993 novella, *Einstein's dreams*, he declares that it is only because our ancestors all die that we are able to live out our lives without their perpetual supervision. Reflecting on the truth of this observation seems to have allowed Hitchens to accept his mortality.

Why has this illness happened to me?

Cosmic responsibility

Four participants canvass what cosmic meaning their prospective deaths might have. Christian believer and clergyman, Mayne, believes that for the cosmos, in the form of God, there is no case to answer: "I don't ask, 'Why me?' .... God could have created a perfect world .... But that would be God's mirror, not his companion, a perversion of the give-and-take of love" (Mayne, p. 50). Atheist Diski has a rather different view, which assumes that if any principle of the universe does exist, it is cruel and arbitrary; she answers a tacit "Why me?" about the suffering caused by the cancer and its treatment with: "It's like a punishment. But for what?" (Diski, p. 208).

For both Hitchens and Taylor, illness and death are random events in a universe indifferent to their fate. According to antitheist Hitchens, to the dim-witted question: "Why me?", the cosmos can barely make the effort to retort with a question of its own: "Why not?" Atheist Taylor reports initially feeling sorry for herself, believing that the universe had cheated her of life that she was entitled to expect, life that would have given her the time to write her *magnum opus;* but over time, her angry response has collapsed into accepting her fate, into a belief that she would be better served if she could just be patient, and bear with her impotence in the face of whatever fate had in store for her. Gould is the only participant for whom the question "Why me"? never comes up; a supreme pragmatist, he initially regards dying as frightening and abhorrent, but soon proceeds to work out how he intends to handle it.

How someone takes being told that they have a terminal illness seems to be related partly to their belief system, and partly to how they receive unmotivated tragic news. Amongst the many different possible responses, four are represented above: first, in our secular modern society, few people regard their oncoming death as of interest to any principle of the universe, and the task facing them may be to find an authentic position from which to accept it; second, for those people who do believe in a personal God, the task facing them may be to find a way to accept his willingness to let them die; third, for those people who already feel weighed down by trauma, the task facing them may be to find a way to understand and forgive themselves and others so as to die in peace, and finally, for those realists for whom dying is yet another, if uniquely formidable event to manage, the task may be to discover which of their remaining concerns matter most, and to choreograph the most fulfilling way to their resolution. For some, the task may involve more than one of these scenarios; for example, Diski is faced with the first and third, and Mayne, with the second and third.

Individual responsibility (i) "I have brought this on myself"

By the age of sixty, Hitchens, Gould and Taylor have all found themselves facing a relatively early death. Indeed, Taylor was merely fifty when first diagnosed with terminal cancer, Gould, fifty-nine and Hitchens, just sixty. Now, it is these same three participants who acknowledge unintentionally and yet, not entirely unwittingly, making themselves vulnerable to developing cancer. By contrast, the two older participants – Mayne and Diski, diagnosed at seventy-five and sixty-seven respectively – might, from their particular medical histories equally have done so, but did not.

Gould was initially diagnosed with advanced and Hitchens, with terminal oesophageal cancer; both believe that their stop-at-nothing, workaholic and hard-living lifestyles had rendered them liable to contracting cancer. Gould locates the beginnings of his digestive tract deterioration in his youth, observing that even then, any stress that he experienced gave him stomach pains. Looking back, he realises that this malaise has never left him; from that time on, gastric pains have become a permanent fixture in his life. Even more careless of his health, Hitchens admits to having worked and socialised early and late, heedlessly risking his well-being until finally, he has been rewarded with an obnoxious little tumour. For both Gould and Hitchens, the cancer represents an alien invader, an opportunist which has seized on their self-neglect as a chance to attack them. As Gould describes it, an uncontrollable tumour is working its way up his gullet like a malevolent alien, while Hitchens, who also refers to the tumour as a malevolent alien, observes drily that while he is constantly being urged to fight it, he can't help thinking that it is the tumour that is making war on him. Nevertheless, on the grounds that their lifestyles had left the door open for it, both Gould and Hitchens blamed themselves for the alien's takeover; and yet, many of their equally high-octane-living colleagues had not fallen prey to cancer. Taylor, the third of this group of self-critics, is dying of a terminal melanoma discovered ten years earlier behind her right knee; for her, the cancer is not so much an invading external alien as the horrendous result of her body generating its destroyer from within. She believes that the melanoma found behind her right knee stemmed from a childhood spent playing in the harsh Queensland sun; at the time, the connection between sun damage and skin cancer had yet to be made. As a more informed adult, however, like Gould and Hitchens, Taylor blames herself for failing to carry out more stringent skin checks; and yet, it is difficult to inspect the skin behind one's knees.

It would appear, then, that all three of these participants were censorious towards themselves for contracting cancer, and were even wondering if they deserved their fate. Indeed, Hitchens suggests that he has actually courted punishment by mocking the Grim Reaper with his risk-taking behaviour. Sounding angry with himself, he follows this verdict with a typically sardonic comment; predictably, he has now had to give way to an illness that is a complete cliché, even to him. His sentiment is echoed by Taylor, who recalls being furious with herself when handed the original diagnosis; in response, she has accused herself of having been too slothful and dumb to bother with skin checks beyond the odd once-over-lightly. Finally, acknowledging that he continued his fast-lane lifestyle against his troubled wife's wishes, Gould believes that the wrong person is being punished. He feels that in letting his wife down, he is the real guilty party. Strikingly, at this stage at least, not one of them expresses any sympathy or concern towards themselves.

Perhaps this state of affairs can be understood as the way these three participants express the obverse side of their customary positive, in-charge approach to life events; even if the outcome has been disastrous, it is *their* outcome, and *they* were its driver. Gould's take on the events so far supports this hypothesis. He reports that strangely enough, for him, the initial diagnosis was actually made more tolerable by the speedy processing of patients into treatment, as this immediately created an atmosphere of hand-to-hand combat with the cancer and therefore, of an objective, and a destination to fight for. On a rather different tack but similarly taking charge, Taylor reports that, filled with horror at how her parents died – bereft of their wits and in institutions – she had determined to do a better job of dying than they had done. Accordingly, she has followed her mother's onetime, but never enacted interest, and has joined the euthanasia-friendly organisation, Exit International. For his part, Hitchens vows to do his utmost to withstand the cancer physically – even if all he can do is to refuse to give way to it – and to secure the best-informed medical help that he can find. Before the cancer struck, in any enterprises that mattered to them, these three participants were used either to taking the lead, or to flying solo, and they appear to have continued to see themselves as prime players even when grappling with forces beyond their control.

Given that today death at sixty-odd is by many considered untimely, it is perhaps no longer reckoned to be 'in the nature of things'; it may be regarded as a death that should not have happened, even as some kind of failure to live well on the part of the deceased. Indeed, Taylor seems to have been under this impression when, railing against the original diagnosis, she laments her failure to catch the cancer at the outset, thus robbing herself of the time she had banked on having to produce her finest work. Arguably, in such cases, both the subject and the world may have come to expect an explanation which would reveal that this prematurely dying person had breached some tacit guidelines for survival. If this is right, for those who believe that some kind of prescription for 'good living' can prevent disease, it might even be thought capable of preventing death itself; if taken seriously, such a mythology would almost certainly have implications for health policy, and for the insurance industry. In addition, it illustrates the emergent proposition that, rather than the truisms about our circumstances which we assume them to be, our beliefs about major life crises like facing death may be strongly influenced by possibly groundless, prevailing contemporary assumptions.

Individual responsibility (ii) "How could this happen to me?"

In contrast with Hitchens, Gould and Taylor, Mayne cannot understand how he contracted cancer. At seventy-five the oldest participant, Mayne is neither a smoker nor a heavy drinker and although he has had it before, he does not think of himself as particularly vulnerable to cancer: "Cancer of the jaw is rare in non-smokers .... Is it connected to the two malignant melanomas of ten years ago? Surely not" (Mayne, pp. 44–45). He describes how he and his dentist jointly delayed his referral to a specialist about a growing oral lump which ultimately turned out to be cancerous: "For months I had had a swelling under my tongue [though] ... X-rays in April showed nothing sinister. But ... an X-ray in June showed an ominous change" (Mayne, p. 45). Similarly, Diski does not seem to connect her cigarette smoking either with her lung cancer or her pulmonary fibrosis. And while she had hoped for more life, she does not rate sixty-eight as being an unduly short life, or her death as particularly untimely. Indeed, as she sees it: "To die pushing seventy years of age is no great tragedy, even if my id would like to know what the fuck age has to do with being rubbed out" (Diski, p. 5). Disdaining to speculate about herself as the cause of her cancer, she refuses to "personify" the cancer cells inside her, rejects "all metaphors of attack or enmity in the midst" – including any reference to "battling with cancer" – and spurns "any notion of desert, punishment, fairness or unfairness or any kind of moral causality" (Diski, p. 10). Unlike Hitchens, Gould and Taylor, she intends to rebut any insinuation that she might have brought the cancer on herself.

There may be many possible reasons for an individual to reject taking some responsibility for failing to prevent cancer from developing. Perhaps Mayne put too much uncritical trust in health professionals, while Diski – perhaps to keep her spirits up – took a pre-emptive stance against any suggestion that she was responsible for becoming ill.

There is another important factor involved in how Mayne and Diski viewed their having contracted cancer; although they led active social lives and were absorbed in their writing activities, they were both past the then commonly-accepted retirement age of sixty-five when diagnosed. Although by no means ready to die, they do not complain that their lives have been unjustly cut short, or ask: "Why me?" about the diagnosis in quite the bitter way that Hitchens and Taylor had done. Further, unlike Hitchens, Taylor and Gould, both Mayne and Diski regard the cancer as having – however inexplicably – arisen naturally from within; to them, it was not due to careless living. Indeed, far from identifying it as an invading alien, it is their intention to establish a relationship with it. As Mayne says: "This is my illness, my cancer, and the form it takes is peculiar to me" (Mayne, p. 50), and: "I seek to give every bit of this new experience my proper attention: to name it, and ... to name the God who is with me in it" (Mayne, p. 58). For Mayne, having cancer is his destiny and part of his God-given life; its good purpose is to be used in the service of himself and others. Diski also sees the cancer as part of herself, but she feels troubled about a lack of support in relating to it. She wishes that she had some recognition and understanding from her oncologist, whom she privately refers to as "Onc Doc": "Everything is presented to me statistically, as probabilities. I can't find the right question to ... talk about the cancer that is me and mine ... how it and I are with each other" (Diski, p. 117). While Mayne can turn to God in making an ongoing relationship with his cancer, Diski feels left alone with an unresponsive doctor, who may be construing her pressing need to know as reason to restrict how much he tells her.

Unlike Gould, Hitchens and Taylor, since they recognise it as an integral part of their own flesh, neither Mayne nor Diski is angry with the cancer as being malevolent or on the attack, nor are they angry with themselves for having developed it. By contrast, although they are profoundly dismayed by its onset, their main concern is to find a way to understand the cancer less as an intruding alien and more – until a way can be found to uproot it – as a known and necessarily tolerated co-habitee.

Why has this happened to me? Summary

Arguably, Mayne and Diski were at diagnosis old enough and by then, far enough away from an everyday working life for the prospect of personal death to have become a part of their subliminal epistemology. On the other hand, for Taylor, Hitchens and Gould – still in the midst of working lives – an implicit awareness of the approach of grave illness may not yet have existed; being identified as host to serious, even terminal cancer, may have been foreign to their here-and-now sense of identity. This is not to suggest that post-retirement brings with it some kind of biologically-based intuitions of mortality. In fact, the joys of an active retirement are widely advertised in our society. At the same time, however, retirement is so construed that it is generally taken to represent the last phase of life; thus, readiness to acknowledge the approach of one's death may be linked more to retirement from working life, than to literal age.

Response to symptomatic warnings

Although every participant had concerning symptoms well before the cancer was actually diagnosed, it is striking that none of them had undertaken early prophylactic action. Hitchens had regularly had toxic morning hangovers and for many years, Gould had had gastric symptoms, yet neither sought an investigation of his symptoms. Taylor wondered why she was not more vigilant about checking her skin, while Mayne acknowledged that for months, he had had a swelling under his tongue which, for too long, dental X-rays had not picked up as cancerous. Finally, pictured on the cover of her memoir with cigarette in hand, Diski had presumably continued as a smoker for some while despite the known connection between smoking and lung cancer, and had already developed pulmonary fibrosis.

Failure to heed advance warnings like these suggests that even those of us who are well-educated and comfortably-off enough to do so, do not necessarily see, take in and apply readily available information about detecting cancer in our bodies. Accordingly, in our health-conscious society, it might be thought that what we need is more information or perhaps, more pressure put on us to undertake investigation of problematic symptoms without delay. Arguably, however, given that in our society, cancer is often taken to be a metaphor for a harrowing death, committing ourselves to the self-surveillance required by cancer checks faces us with a cruel dilemma. On the one hand, we are responsible for maintaining a healthy lifestyle and for regularly checking ourselves out. On the other, our very own explorations might hand us a death sentence. Indeed, the best we can hope for with cancer checks is – *this time* – not to find anything. Diski's cancer was found at a routine screening of her pulmonary fibrosis; she had not sought, and did not reckon on its also revealing a diagnosis of lung cancer. Accidental discoveries aside, however, any of us might, like Taylor, shrink from being scrupulous about regular skin-examinations or like Gould, Hitchens, and Mayne, postpone for too long an investigation of a symptom which, perhaps as one amongst several, we have deemed to be innocuous, and accustomed ourselves to tolerating.

Response to symptomatic warnings: Summary

Arguably, it is *because* we have become so sensitised to cancer as a prelude to death that when we are on the verge of detecting possible signs or symptoms of it, our fear that it may already be too late to save ourselves may blind us to them. As is further discussed in Chapter 8, *Themes in the experience of dying*, it may be time for the healthcare managements of advanced societies to review the effectiveness of self-reporting assessments in their policies and programs, and to consider the possibility of instead including them in regular check-ups done by health professionals.

Emotional responses

All participants wrote extensively in this category.

Participants' immediate emotional responses to receiving a cancer diagnosis

There is a wide variety in the immediate responses the participants record to receiving their initial cancer diagnosis. Having received her terminal diagnosis ten years previously, Taylor's feelings of terror and anguish at the time have by now diminished; she has become more composed, and her feelings of anxiety about dying are only intermittent. On the other hand, regret about the independence and mobility she has lost over the years is becoming increasingly prominent; she can no longer drive a car, or enjoy their once daily walks by the river with her husband. In effect, she is now confined to two rooms of her home, her bedroom and the living room. What she most laments, however, is finding that, apart from her peers at Exit International, talking about personal death is excluded from everyday conversation; she believes the dying have probably never been more lonely.

Even though for Mayne and Gould the initial diagnosis was not terminal, as it was for Taylor, Hitchens and Diski – that came later – they were both initially overcome with shock and dread, and left struggling for composure. Following his first, though not yet terminal diagnosis, Gould describes waking up that night in the grip of alarm and consternation, attacked from all sides by demonic dark thoughts. Identifying what was really troubling him – one of his most useful skills – he says that it is not so much what lies ahead that dismays him, it is its inevitability. Immediately, through finding ways to control them, he sets out to eliminate the fear of being overwhelmed by his feelings. His regimen for developing what he calls 'basic cancer survival skills' includes developing the ability to change his mood at will, to hear, and yet not hear, any bad news, and generally, to turn negatives into positives. Arguably, Gould's many years in leading political campaigns have taught him a variety of techniques in self-management, and before long, his natural ebullience returns. Just as he has found in so many elections, he begins to feel optimistic and excited, convinced once more that against all odds, he will prevail. Sustained by this view, he doesn't report a lasting adverse reaction to being given bad news until a third and terminal diagnosis cuts right through his defences. Although he has never thought of himself as especially emotional, with death suddenly only three months away, he finds himself overwhelmed with distress. Looking at Gail (his wife), he bursts into tears; never in his life has he talked to her with such intensity.

On receiving his first, also not yet terminal, diagnosis, Mayne's fear and distress about what might happen to him remains for some time undiminished. Half of his entries in this category concern the suffering the diagnosis and prospective treatment are causing him: "The reality hits you afresh each day on waking .... Moments of panic and mild nausea" (Mayne, p. 46); "[I feel] ... concern for A. [his wife, Alison] and the family, the stress they will be under .... the fear of feverish dreams and nightmares .... [W]hat about pain control?" (Mayne, pp. 50–51); "[O]ccasionally, the heart lurches as the imagination unhelpfully explores the unpredictable" (Mayne, p. 47). He attempts to steady himself, with mixed results: "One part of me is immature and panicky, the other mature and in control .... Meanwhile, I believe this cancer will be cured" (Mayne, p. 51). But despite its being thought to be treatable, the cancer diagnosis has also made him think about dying: "When cancer is diagnosed .... It is a tap on the shoulder ... a ...reminder of your mortality" (Mayne, p. 169). He reproaches himself for being self-centred, perhaps to shake off his anxiety and 'man up': "Ashamed to be self-obsessed on a terrible day of bombs on London Underground" (Mayne, p. 47). Other entries refer to his struggles to find support in his faith in God: "'Thou wilt keep him in perfect peace, whose mind has stayed on thee.' Yes: but at times the mind refuses to be stayed" (Mayne, p. 46). Ultimately, it is the thought of the people who have offered him solace that most comforts him now: "There is a steady sense of being held and encouraged by many expressions of loving support" (Mayne, p. 58), and as with Gould, it is the idea of the loss of the relationship with his wife that most saddens him: "If ... one should die, there is no greater anguish ... [than having] no one to share the intimacies of your life" (Mayne, p. 124).

While for some time, Mayne finds himself almost inconsolable in the face of the initial diagnosis, Gould soon recovers; naturally ebullient, he has also mastered a set of techniques for managing potentially overwhelming emotions. Indeed, Gould's ability to maintain a positive attitude remains formidable up to his last breath. By contrast, the gentle and deeply-feeling Mayne has to find within himself the spiritual and emotional strength to endure the anxiety with no ready-made strategies to ease the pain.

In complete contrast with Mayne, Gould and Taylor, Diski and Hitchens withdraw into emotional distancing and avoidance; they fend off anxiety by deploying a distant, even satirical attitude to receiving their diagnoses. More than half of Hitchens' initial reactions are not overtly emotional; rather, they are almost brutally down-to-earth. Early on, he issues instructions to himself: leaving the good times and spontaneity of his previous life behind, he must instead maintain a constant and onerous mindfulness about his present circumstances. At the same time, however, he absolutely rejects, as the ultimate banality, being described as 'fighting cancer'. Moreover, although he experiences sadness about his lost future – for example, about not being there to see his children marry – he determines that he will never indulge in being pathetic and feeling sorry for himself, and he will not allow other people to access his vulnerabilities either. Indeed, he recoils when offered sympathy, wishing that he could ban all such verbal intrusions. Finally, despite its making him feel engulfed in something toxic and, into the bargain, depriving him of his sexual function, he is prepared to accept chemotherapy and any other treatment that is offered to him.

Taking the theme of ennui much further than Hitchens does, Diski's initial response to the diagnosis seems counter-intuitive. Her immediate reaction epitomises it: "The future flashed before my eyes in all its preordained banality" (Diski, p.1). At first, she experiences embarrassment, along with: "a weariness [as] ... when you are set on track by something outside your control ... [But] you could ... jot down ... every single thing that will happen" (Diski, p. 1). Then, finding herself wondering how long she has to live, she reports: "I was mortified ... that ... I was already a predictable cancer patient" (Diski, p. 2), and: "The great weariness ... at the idea of asking [how long?] … and setting the expected ball of clichés rolling, was overwhelming" (Diski, pp. 3–4).

Eventually becoming angry, Diski has fantasies of punishing the doctor: "Do I want to ask that obvious next question? …. (How long, then, without treatment?) …. Why should I make it easy for him?" (Diski, p. 3); "I could … sit in sadistic silence waiting for whatever is next on his list of diagnostic appointment moves …. 'Yes? And?'" (Diski, p. 4), and finally – in imitation of Jack Lemmon, sticking her neck out, and yelling in "Onc Doc's" face: "'You're telling me I've got CANCER? …. I'm going to be DEAD IN THREE YEARS. If I'm LUCKY. Have I got that RIGHT?'" (Diski, pp 4–5). In fact, out of nine entries, there are only two which register shock and anxiety, both about wondering how long she has to live:

> [It] suddenly struck me … that [weeks] … could be his answer …. Every cell in my body began lindy-hopping …. With … 'to treat, not to cure'… [Onc Doc] … had told me that I was going to die … sooner rather than later
>
> (Diski, pp. 2–3)

and: "This not crazily short but vague two-to-three years is a difficult real life calculation for me" (Diski, p. 5).

It is not hard to understand that someone who has just been given an unexpected death sentence might feel like shooting the messenger. However, it is striking that Diski registers fear and shock at her tragic news just twice, while six of her nine entries emphasise her overwhelming feelings of embarrassment and weariness, interspersed with sadistic fantasies directed at the oncologist. It is possible that the weariness is partly the result of shock at an unexpected diagnosis; further, she has rapidly assessed what lies ahead, a debilitating prospect. But it is more difficult to assign a plausible explanation for her being flooded with embarrassment, and she does not offer one. Is it due to what she has been told, or more likely, to how she construes the position she now occupies in relation to the doctor-nurse couple? When handed the diagnosis, Diski had made a satirical joke about "cooking the meth" – making drugs – and the doctor showed no sign that he had even heard her speak (Diski, p. 1). For someone as hypersensitive to rebuff as Diski turns out to be, having her banter ignored by the oncologist would be profoundly galling. Arguably, since she then rapidly concludes that this doctor who has the power of life and death over her uses pre-set interview scripts and treats his patients as items on a running agenda, it could seem to her humiliating, even degrading, to go cap in hand to ask him how long she has to live. If this is right, what she calls feeling embarrassment at receiving the diagnosis might, more appropriately, be called feeling shamed. Again, Diski also shows minimal solicitude towards herself in the face of calamity; in her epistemology, compassion towards herself does not seem to exist.

Diski's entries so far appear to be generally unlike those of the other participants. However, there is some common ground between Diski and Hitchens; for Diski, finding her role in a trite cancer narrative wearisome and predictable sounds similar to Hitchens finding his boring and banal, and they both detest being described as 'battling with cancer'.

Participants' immediate emotional responses to receiving a cancer diagnosis: Summary

Gould, Hitchens and Mayne – unlike Diski – were all broadly positive about their oncologists' approach to their illness and plans for treatment; by now, Taylor's treatment regimen was well-established, and she seldom mentions it. While Gould felt badly about ignoring his wife's protests about his lifestyle – as did Taylor about failing to contact Exit International to help her mother to die, when she was institutionalised – guilt about failing someone over a specific issue is quite distinct from the embarrassment or shame expressed by Diski; shame is a more global and archaic emotion, directed against the self as being intrinsically unacceptable. And although Mayne expressed shame about his reaction of self-absorbed misery, his emotion was more like guilt – feeling badly about being so preoccupied with his own misfortune when that of others was so much worse. What might have motivated Diski's atypical reaction to the initial diagnosis is examined in depth in Chapter 7, *Acceptance*.

Analysis of participants' emotional responses

All participants feel stress about having cancer *per se*, although they deal with it differently. They all fear the loss of control that awaits them – control over their emotions, their affairs, their bodies and their independence. As seen above, Gould, Hitchens and Mayne are all distressed about the inescapable physical suffering associated with cancer and its treatment; Hitchens is also afraid of losing control of his emotions. Diski's fears about bodily collapse are realistic: "I will be fighting for breath with both [diseases]…" (Diski, p.154), while Taylor is sufficiently frightened of becoming helpless that for some time, she has had thoughts of euthanising herself. Finally, all participants are overcome by grief at the prospective loss of their spouse and immediate family. For Diski, this grieving is also focused on the loss of her infant grandchildren: "I feel the sadness even more sharply, now that the new girl child has been born, at the idea of missing knowing what they will both be like" (Diski, p.156).

Noted earlier by Elias (1985) as a widespread phenomenon facing the dying, Taylor does stress her experiences of its loneliness. She observes that, apart from her colleagues in Exit International meetings, people distance themselves from the dying, and avoid talking about it. And although Mayne does not himself complain about suffering from the pain of becoming isolated, he emphasises in his memoir that he hopes to alleviate it in others.

None of the other participants mentions being avoided by other people, or feeling isolated or lonely. Therefore, as noted in Chapter 3. Part II, no significant support for Elias' depiction of the loneliness of the dying is provided by the participants in this study; however, in the strength of their connectedness with others, they may not be typical of the wider society

Four participants express distress about causing anxiety to their families – as seen above, Mayne and Gould are distressed for their wives; Diski is troubled about her husband's grief: "When the Poet expresses his sadness and forthcoming grief, it hits me as if I were him suffering his loss of me" (Diski, p. 142), and Taylor, about how much strain the ups and downs of her long time dying is putting on her family. A slightly different group of four participants is afflicted by the harshness of the treatment – Gould, Mayne and Hitchens as above, and Diski, who has become unable to tolerate the chemotherapy drugs. Taylor is the only participant to say little about treatment; after ten years as a cancer patient, her treatment appears to be an established regimen. Three participants mention losing much-loved activities – some of them central to their sense of self – from everyday living: Taylor's daily walks by the river with her husband are over; Diski mourns the passing of her consuming interest: "'What's the point?' Only earning my living by writing" (Diski, p. 213), and Hitchens fears that the treatment is causing his self-identity to dissipate, that his very personality is dissolving as his hands become numb, threatening to leave his thoughts forever unrecorded. By contrast, however, two participants feel that, despite the losses of so many normal enjoyments, a worthwhile quality of life can still be maintained. According to Mayne: "These last days [are about] ... not the *amount* of time left to me but its *quality*" (Mayne, p. 246), while Gould experiences his dying as a time full of ecstatic moments and unparalleled fulfilment, in which he has enjoyed the closest of relationships with all of his family.

Resources used by participants to deal with emotional distress

During these times of hardship, every participant seeks support from external sources. All participants turn to their spouses, family and friends; Diski to her husband and daughter, and Mayne to his wife, his family and his circle of friends: "There is a steady sense of being held and encouraged by many expressions of loving support" (Mayne, p. 58); for Gould, it is his family who have made it possible for him to survive this ordeal, and for Hitchens, it is his conversation-loving, attentive friends; finally, for Taylor, perhaps because it is less stressful for all parties, communication is most open and free with her cheerful, and at times blackly humorous, Exit International group, rather than with her caring family. The two Christian participants also seek help from God. Initially, Mayne felt out of touch with him but as the illness progresses, he reveals that: "What I have learned is that, while God may often seem remote ... yet .... God's grace works through the kindness [of] ... people whose lives we have touched" (Mayne, p. 245). For Gould, the opposite trend takes place; as the cancer progresses, the part his faith plays in his life diminishes. Now close to suffering and death, he has found that, just at the critical moment when he most needs it, his once reliable faith has failed him; however, this has allowed his faith to move to a different place, making room for the kind of questioning and doubting that is better matched to his personality.

For all participants, finding ways to manage distress and worry has high priority, and although for different reasons, Mayne and Hitchens share a determination to shut down self-pity, the resources accessed by the participants are otherwise all different. By the end of his life, Mayne draws strength directly from his relationship with God: "I find myself saying more and more: 'I can do all things through Christ who strengthens me'" (Mayne, pp. 248–249). An expert in mind-games, Gould has resorted to a number of acquired techniques he can deploy to turn away threatening ideas. For example, he first developed the habit of treating his fears like a video game, turning away each negative pressure as it came, and eventually, of simply resorting to straight up self-affirmations. In the end, he learnt how to alter his mood at will, an ability he believes to be basic to surviving cancer. For Hitchens, there is distraction and sustenance in contacts with friends, and in public debating, and he continues to seize every chance that he can to participate in verbal jousting matches. For a time, Diski finds refuge in an idea which is reminiscent of Lucretius' argument against fearing death: "I have been *not here* before .... I have already been absent, non-existent .... This thought is ... the only one that works, to calm me down when the panic comes" (Diski, pp. 149–150). She also turns to professional carers: "I'm ... seeing a counsellor once a week who has spent ten years ... getting people ready for death" (Diski, p. 211). Finally, writing her memoir has from the outset been sustaining for her. As reported, Taylor finds the loneliness of modern dying painful, but her Exit group is supportive.

Two participants – Diski and Hitchens – share an aversion to being subjected to banal descriptions like 'battling cancer'. It might seem that they are being irritably precious about not very much; however, it may rather be that they are worried about being tagged with platitudes because their status as cancer patients could make other people try to avoid more personal contact with them. If this is right, it must be asked if other participants share the same concern about preserving their individuality, though perhaps differently expressed? Arguably, they all do. For example, Mayne and Gould both emphasise the need for authenticity before social correctness; for Mayne: "In the end, books are about ... what matters to us most, our desire to 'speak what we feel, not what we ought to say'" (Mayne, pp. 245–246), while for Gould, knowing that others might not agree with what he wrote changed nothing; he would do it all again. And in concentrating on telling the reader something meaningful about herself and what her dying is like before she dies, Taylor is clearly intent upon providing an account of her genuine self. Discovering that even medical professionals and certainly other people generally find it hard to relate to sufferers from an archetypal scourge like cancer, a cancer patient may develop a fear of being bypassed as an individual and instead, identified and distanced by the use of medical labels and trite phrases. If this is right, such a concern is probably more widespread than we realise. For all the participants in this study, the need to be identified as an individual at the last is urgent; recognition of this need by healthcare professionals may not only enhance patients' relationships with them but also, boost their compliance with treatment.

Analysis of participants' emotional responses: Summary

Six areas of emotional concern were highly important to all participants – having cancer *per se*; the prospect of parting from their spouses and families; the potential loss of control of everything important in their lives; having the support of family and friends, medical carers and others; finding the resources in the self and in the community to manage painful feelings and finally, needing to maintain their individuality and to have it recognised by others. Three further issues were significant to a majority of participants – for four participants, Mayne, Gould, Taylor and Diski, causing stress and grief to the spouse and family, and distress about the treatment were important, while three participants – Taylor, Diski and Hitchens – emphasised the loss of enjoyable pursuits and quality of life in general. Although referred to as important by only two participants – Mayne and Gould – two further items should be mentioned: Firstly, that a worthwhile quality of life can be maintained by dedicated effort and secondly, that while in the midst of suffering and distress, religious believers may feel that their God seems remote from their present traumatic condition, reviewing their relationship with their faith can give rise to an outcome that is authentic and satisfying.

Arguably, the study shows that there is no more or less resilient way of responding to a cancer diagnosis, whether terminal or not. Rather, even though the study has only five participants, the themes emerging from their emotional responses illustrate the range of emotional work required of them, and their perseverance and resourcefulness in addressing it. However, for those who cannot access support themselves, as will be seen in Chapter 8, *Themes in the experience of dying*, there are specialised programs available which can benefit the dying in general, and cancer patients in particular.

Does facing cancer equate with facing death?

For Taylor, Diski and Hitchens, the cancer diagnosis is terminal from the outset, while for both Mayne and Gould, the terminal diagnosis only came some two years after an initially more optimistic diagnosis and much investment in treatment. From the start, however, Mayne vacillates between the fear of dying and hopes of survival. Referring to Shakespeare's tragic protagonist, Mayne quotes from Hamlet's intimations of death, immediately followed by attempts to reassure himself that his own and Hamlet's cases are not the same: "The words ... keep coming to mind .... [of] Hamlet's 'The readiness is all'.... Meanwhile, I believe this cancer will be cured" (Mayne, p. 51). Gould was also terrified by the initial diagnosis, but his work on remaining positive has borne fruit; even after the cancer's recurrence, he remains optimistic of a substantial remission, and is therefore determined to see a second major operation through. Of the three participants who received a terminal diagnosis at the outset – Taylor, Hitchens and Diski – neither Hitchens nor Diski records more than a passing feeling of anxiety initially though ten years later, Taylor reports having been frightened and distressed by receiving the diagnosis. At the time of writing the memoir, however, her fears are no longer of dying *per se*, but of a prolonged period of what she imagines as being a bad way to die. For Hitchens and Diski, the apprehension caused by the terminal diagnosis is not so much absent as delayed. Sometime after the diagnosis, Diski becomes persistently anxious about dying: "Whatever terror there is lies in the present fear of dying, not so much of death" (Diski, p. 162). Hitchens' anxiety is not so much about dying itself, as of dying in a delusional state due to the effects of the chemotherapy on his brain; he is afraid that he will become unable to distinguish dying under hospital protocols from being subjected to elaborate torture, to be followed by a sadistic execution. In the more immediate future, he dreads the possibility that in damaging his ability to communicate, the treatment is already causing him to face the onset of a living death.

Of the two participants who did not initially receive a terminal diagnosis, Mayne nonetheless reports persisting high levels of anxiety in the weeks following diagnosis; by contrast, Gould dispatches his terrors in days, and until receiving his terminal diagnosis two years later, maintains his expectation of becoming cancer-free. Once terminally ill, however, he is initially anxious about how frighteningly close dying might be. Never one to gloss over ugly facts, he reflects on his now drastically reduced future; in no more than six weeks, he will be dead, and in the meantime, whenever his symptoms spiral out of control, he will face terror. And while Mayne also hopes for some time that his cancer will be cured, he still regards the diagnosis as a reminder of his mortality, and acknowledges that he fears dying: "Fear of the dark and the unknown are common to us all" (Mayne, p. 92).

Combined with the particular trajectory of their illness, the nature, degree and timing of the participants' anxieties are characteristic of them as individuals. For all participants, however, their fears are focused on two areas. Firstly, there is the fear associated with having cancer and the effects of the treatment, and secondly, there is the fear of dying, due either to enduring a horrible death, or to being thrust alone, and somehow still conscious, into the unknown, or both. In fact, these perilous contingencies appear to concern the participants more than the prospect of death itself. Actually, as discussed in Chapter 2, *Death as enigma*, none of the participants appears to be able to conceptualise their own death *per se*, or therefore, to be capable of identifying a response to it.

Does facing cancer equate with facing death? Summary

Ultimately, it is not clear whether the participants' foremost concern relates to living with cancer and enduring the treatment, or to dying from it; certainly, once terminally diagnosed, these factors are inextricably intertwined for them all. While the present-day availability of heart bypass surgery, stents and pacemakers have enabled many sufferers from potentially deadly heart problems to be restored to health and longer life, cancer is the disease *par excellence* from which it is widely understood that true recovery cannot be relied on; the best hope still appears to be a 'worthwhile remission'. Arguably, whether or not the original cancer diagnosis carries a death sentence, in our society cancer is still widely regarded as its harbinger.

Terminal versus non-terminal diagnosis: Effect on participant's emotional response

It might be expected that the entries of the participants who received terminal diagnoses at the outset – Diski, Hitchens and Taylor – would show more anxiety or stronger emotional reactions to the diagnosis than those of Mayne and Gould, who did not receive theirs until two years later. As noted above, ten years on from diagnosis, Taylor's feelings about dying of cancer have become relatively composed, while Diski and Hitchens both distance themselves on first receiving a terminal diagnosis. Diski does not become agitated about death or dying until later, while Hitchens never allows anything to undermine his gladiatorial stance towards the cancer for long. By contrast, although Mayne's prognosis remains positive until only about three months before his death, the initial diagnosis leaves him full of foreboding regarding the cancer's threat to his quality of life and indeed, to life itself. Gould also first reacts to the cancer diagnosis with terror but unlike Mayne, he is accomplished in manipulating his emotions; accordingly, the terror is soon dispatched, and until he receives his terminal diagnosis, his only moderately justified confidence about defeating the cancer returns.

Excluding Taylor in this case because her reaction to her initial diagnosis was not recorded at the time, the participants' emotional responses to the diagnosis appear to be individually determined. It is notable that Mayne and Gould – who received non-terminal diagnoses – were initially more thrown off balance than were Diski and Hitchens, who received terminal diagnoses at the outset. This is hard to understand if being given a non-terminal diagnosis is regarded as similar to, but less confronting, than being given a terminal diagnosis. In fact, however, the two types of diagnosis offer quite different, but comparably daunting, challenges to their recipients.

Both Mayne and Gould had major cancers, the treatment of which they were told at diagnosis would make formidable demands on them. For Gould, the first surgery on offer proposed breaking his ribs and entering his stomach and upper chest by major incision, after which the large tumour and any ancillaries would be removed. Unsurprisingly, when reporting on his second though not yet terminal cancer diagnosis, Gould is unenthusiastic about the proposed second surgery. Rather, he is inclined to bargain, to ask how much longer he will live if he has the surgery; on the surgeon's reply that it would probably be six months to a year, he does opt for the surgery, to buy more time. For Mayne, surgery would take place in his neck and several parts of his mouth, and the excised areas would be reconstructed from flaps of flesh from his thigh. Reflecting on this prospective treatment causes Mayne anguish: "My anxieties are [about] … the fear of feverish dreams and nightmares …. Will I be able to speak properly again? Will I lose my sense of taste and smell? *All* my teeth? And what about pain control?" (Mayne, pp. 50–51). Both were to spend twelve hours in theatre, endure extreme pain and suffer from drug-induced hallucinations. Further, both would later have to undergo chemotherapy and possibly, radiation therapy. By contrast, as their cancers were inoperable, the only treatment proposed for Diski and Hitchens was to be chemotherapy and radiation. Taylor has had brain surgery to improve her quality of life just prior to writing her memoir, and did not refer to having any significant treatment after that.

Terminal versus non-terminal diagnosis: Effect on participant's emotional response: Summary

Receiving a death sentence at initial diagnosis is like being poleaxed – it would be hard at first for those participants suddenly facing death to think clearly or grasp their imminent death as a reality. By contrast, an excruciating treatment regimen prescribed as a condition of survival may be only too easy to imagine, and once heard, impossible to forget. In fact, quite different, but equally intense demands are made on their recipients by these diagnoses. Suddenly faced with having no future, the recipient of a terminal diagnosis is left stunned; on the other hand, a non-terminal diagnosis sends its recipient on a grim journey of indeterminate length, to an uncertain destination. Either way, their experience is traumatic; there will be much to endure, and their lives will be changed forever.

How long do I have?

The question of how much life was predicted to be left to them might be expected to elicit a spate of attempts at bargaining from the participants.

More life or better quality of life?

On receiving a terminal diagnosis and after suffering many months of harrowing treatment, Mayne decides that further chemotherapy would be for dubious gain: "These last days [are about] … not the *amount* of time left to me but its *quality*" (Mayne, p. 246). By now post-treatment, Taylor focuses only on quality of life; she has her euthanasia drug to fall back on if her condition deteriorates too far into helplessness. For Hitchens, however, all life is worth having; he has committed himself to meeting whatever the cancer thrusts upon him, and although he knows that his illness is bound to get worse, he intends to stay the course as far as he can. And when Gould's diagnosis becomes terminal, like Mayne, he is told the truth; despite two major surgeries, his life is now almost over. Knowing that he will not survive more than three months, he is terse; as he sees it, he and his doctors are orchestrating the management of his death. Unlike Mayne and Taylor, for Hitchens and Gould, more life invariably emerges as the prime *desideratum*; however, once the game is up, they both recognise it.

Subject to a terminal diagnosis from the outset, Diski is frustrated by the vagueness of her prognosis: "To be told that with an effort I might live for another two or three years brought back the uncertainty .... Can I learn to live with certain uncertainty, or uncertain certainty?" (Diski, pp. 138–139). As the waiting drags on, however, Diski does finally consider a bargaining proposition: "A decline caused by fibrosis or lung cancer is very unpleasant. But ... the prospect of stronger and nastier medication, left me thinking about the balance .... [Q]uality of life .... Versus, I suppose, no life at all" (Diski, pp. 160–161); adrift in a sea of imponderables, she seems to remain irresolute.

More life or better quality of life: Summary

As is probably typical of cancer sufferers, for the four participants whose prognoses are by now well-defined – Gould, Hitchens, Mayne and Taylor – bargaining of only one kind is evident; the value of compliance with harsh treatment is regularly set against time to be gained from undergoing it. However, if submitting to treatment will damage its quality, acquiring more time is not always going to be preferred.

The problem of the asymptomatic terminal diagnosis

As noted above, owing to the history and advanced state of their illness, at terminal diagnosis, the prognoses of Hitchens, Gould, Mayne and Taylor could be relatively well-defined; moreover, they actually felt mortally ill. For Diski, however, the tumour was only an image on a scan; in addition, the initial prognosis of possibly two to three years seemed to her so vague that any increases in it for compliance with treatment or subtractions from it for the opposite, would probably seem equally meaningless. After eighteen months of treatment, she describes her predicament: "With the new drugs, if they work on me – 'perhaps a year'.... I don't exactly feel ill now. I'm trapped in a mesh of steroid effects" (Diski, p. 208). Given that the radiation therapy had rendered her pulmonary fibrosis suffocating and terminal, for Diski, the treatment side effects had become the illness and the illness itself remained a chimera; compliance with treatment therefore became a major challenge.

Near the end of her memoir, she is approaching a final decision: "I've been given one last chance. A trial pill .... The last lot I stopped because they made me sick .... These new ones have bad side-effects after which there is 'nothing we can do for you'" (Diski, p. 245). What she decided to do is not recorded, but she might well have concluded that there could be no deal. In fact, she died a few weeks after making the above entry, three months short of the minimum two years estimated in her original prognosis.

There are two significant clinical problems associated with asymptomatic terminal diagnoses; the first of these is seen when a patient experiences *radical disbelief*. Due to the diagnostic capacities of modern medical technology people who, like Diski, are not even aware that they have cancer, can unexpectedly be confronted at routine examinations by evidence that they are already dying from it. Arguably, for these individuals, an abyss is opened up between the terminal diagnosis and their sense of being-in-life which creates a response not so much of denial of the diagnosis, as of a state of mind prior to this: a state of radical disbelief. That is, as in my own experience, the diagnosis has been heard, but has not resonated and been taken in. It might be argued that as I did not have metastatic lung cancer, my disbelief was based on fact, but because I did not actually dispute the diagnosis, it would be hard to mount a cogent argument to that effect. To be in a state of radical disbelief does not imply that its recipient believes that the diagnosis is *wrong*; that would be to disagree with it. Rather, the diagnosis is accepted as correct, but because its recipient does not experience any matching sense of impairment, it may not be possible for them to take it on board. Arguably, until the condition identified by the terminal illness is experienced as part of someone's being-in-life, it cannot become part of that individual's psychic reality. If this is right, Diski's pleas to be helped to relate to the cancer and it to her might be understood as an appeal to her oncologist for help in grasping what she never denied, but could not experience as true. Diski laments this deprivation of realness: "Everything is presented to me statistically, as probabilities. I can't find the right question to ... talk about the cancer that is me and mine ... how it and I are with each other" (Diski, p. 117). In fact, until the end of her life, Diski still experiences a disconnect between the diagnosis, the treatment, and her sense of being-in-life: "What could anyone give me that could definitively improve my health? .... [W]hen most of the unwellnesss came from the treatment?" (Diski, p. 207).

Being in a state of radical disbelief has to be distinguished from being 'in denial' about death or dying. Being in denial refers to the failure to acknowledge the reality of human death in general, or of one's own in particular, or both. According to social psychologist Camilla Zimmermann, it is becoming accepted in modern society that being open to conversation about one's dying and death is a way into a 'good death'; certainly, it is valued by health professionals as a means to discussing with a patient important issues like Advance Care Planning, and the cessation of futile treatments. By contrast, failure to communicate about one's approaching death can be construed as being 'in denial' and accordingly, seen as an obstacle to a 'good death' (Zimmermann, 2007, p. 297). Given that Zimmermann bases her observations on thirty articles on best practice in palliative care, it seems likely that 'important discussions' and 'good deaths' are constructs created by the specialist medical professionals involved, rather than by the dying themselves.

Social scientist Alex Broom confirms this view: "The discourse on acceptance and the denial-acceptance dichotomy sustains an ideal of a preferred way to die" (Broom, 2012, p. 223). Further, hospital physician Tara Tucker claims that the routine misdiagnosis and dismissal of the reticent dying as being 'in denial' is in effect professionally negligent (Tucker, 2009). Moreover, what clinicians in this case are calling 'being in denial' does not distinguish between true denial – an involuntary unconscious defence mechanism, which it is impossible voluntarily to set aside in the interests of discussing 'important issues' – and choosing not to speak, which may, for example, be due to natural reserve, or to a fear of giving control of the situation to some as yet untried medical professional. Either way, in dismissing a patient's failure to communicate as their 'being in denial', clinicians could be failing to distinguish true denial from patient reticence and moreover, construing both states as quasi-clinical syndromes of intentional non-co-operation.

Accordingly, being in a state of radical disbelief is both different from, and prior to, being in denial and therefore, the medical response to seemingly uncooperative patients does need to be calibrated with care. Without this, it is possible that a patient's condition of experiential disconnect from their illness will be mistaken for 'being in denial'; their treating professionals may remonstrate with them or, believing that the patient has closed down, withdraw their interest. For example, while in my own state of radical disbelief, I was seen at my GP clinic by a doctor whom I did not know to discuss some recent CT scan results. When I appeared pleased that no tumour had been found, he drove his chair across the room to confront me and raising his voice, declared: "You should be hoping that we find the primary! You're just afraid of dying!" Mercifully, I found another GP with whom I could discuss my dilemma. Unfortunately, however, like Diski, many terminally ill people in a state of disconnect may miss out on the benefits of an experiential awareness of their condition which, if they had understood the problem, their medical professionals might have been able to help them to recognise. Given that tolerating harsh treatment depends on a whole-hearted commitment to wrestle with having cancer, an unrecognised state of radical disbelief is likely to lead to wasted treatment and truncated lives in the way that it did for Diski. In contrast with her, and afflicted by periods of increasingly severe illness, the other participants had good existential reason to tolerate distressing treatments and ultimately, also knew when it was time to stop doing so, and to prepare themselves to die.

The second clinical problem can be seen when a patient is given a prognosis based on statistical probability rather than on their own particular condition; the patient may experience the loss of a sense of agency. As was deplored by

Diski, it is likely to become more common in our society for the terminally-ill to find that their prognoses are based primarily on the statistical probabilities clinical research assigns to their condition. Arguably, as an item in a demographic cohort, they are liable to be exposed more to uncertainty and the loss of a sense of agency than someone whose prognosis and treatment are tailored more directly to their experienced condition. If this is right, some people facing death may have to live with a known to be foreshortened and yet, indeterminate future; for them, an unrecognised and stressful limbo may open up between the diagnosis and the final illness.

In recognition of the suffering of patients who do feel that they have to wait too long to die, the Victorian government directed the Legislative Council to investigate current end-life-care; in 2017, this resulted in legislation which allows some of the terminally ill to access assisted dying from doctors if their pain and suffering cannot be sufficiently alleviated (Anderson, 2017, p. 1). It is not clear yet how many Victorians will make use of the legislation but typically, it is a very small group. For example, in the state of Washington in the USA, only 240 people chose to make use of newly-available physician-assisted dying in the period from 2009 to the end of 2012 (Health research funding, 2014, para. 18). Accordingly, it has been argued that other populations besides the terminally ill could appropriately be included in the legislation – for example, those who suffer from chronic diseases and have little quality of life (Hutchinson, 2017, p. 12). Indeed, between 2000 and 2013, of the more than 170,000 people living in nursing homes across Australia, 140 took their own lives; 70% of these were isolated men, and 66% had a diagnosis of depression. Their problems included loneliness, feelings of being cut-off, and chronic health deterioration (Murphy and Ibrahim, 2018, paras. 1, 2, 5 and 6).

It is not being suggested that the condition of the anomie-afflicted terminally ill is coterminous with despairing nursing home populations, but they have in common features like poor health and decreased quality of life; both are also vulnerable to being cut off from the purposeful hum of everyday living or even, as Gould put it, from the heartening sense of the struggle, purpose and endpoint generated by an active treatment regimen. Diski's feeling of having been abandoned as recalcitrant by the medical world shows how having little meaningful communication with medical professionals about her treatment, together with having no sense of agency about the terms of her life expectancy, could have exposed her to developing feelings of futility. From there, it may only be a short distance to giving up the struggle to go on living. As Diski put it: "I've been feeling as if I'm on a holiday, a short one coming to its end. Not an especially good one" (Diski, p. 246).

How long do I have? Summary

Facing death in the foreseeable future involves the task of preparing to die; what is required for this work is discussed in the next two chapters. For those immobilised by a state of radical disbelief, or exposed to uncertainty about their future and the loss of a sense of agency, however, there may be no real-time sense of how far ahead their lives will extend. If the ambiguity of their position is pervasive enough, they may be unable to access the necessary psychological resources within themselves to prepare for dying; as well as appropriately sensitive medical responsiveness, such individuals may need therapeutic help, whether mentoring or counselling.

Part III. Cancer as part of the self (*Is the cancer seen as part of the self? Does accepting cancer as part of the self lead to a 'better' death?*)

All participants express an opinion about this issue.

Is the cancer seen as part of the self?

Diski, Mayne and Taylor believe that their cancer has emerged from within and is therefore an integral, if destructive, part of themselves. According to Diski: "I [need] … to talk about the cancer that is me and mine" (Diski, p. 117); to Mayne: "This is my illness, my cancer, and the form it takes is peculiar to me" (Mayne, p. 50); Taylor also believes that the cancer has arisen from within, and although acknowledging that it was over-exposed to the sun's rays in her childhood, she feels that in becoming cancerous, her body has engineered its own destruction. On the other hand, Gould and Hitchens both see the cancer as a foreign invader to be fought off. From the outset, Hitchens has intended to combat the cancer with all his strength, while Gould's equally determined resistance to it has drawn additional strength from his oncologist's support; as he describes it, his consultant is ready to join him in fighting to the end. By contrast, Diski probably, and as is seen in the next chapter, Mayne definitely, reject treatment some weeks before death, because they feel that its side-effects will destroy whatever quality of life remains to them.

For Gould and Hitchens, plugging into all treatments is the highway to maintaining the struggle against the alien invader. In essence, they understand that in this context, what is good and worth saving is internal to them, and what is bad and destructive is external. By contrast, Diski and Mayne understand that human beings are made up of destructive as well as positive characteristics and accordingly, they can accept the cancer as an integral part of themselves. For them, quality of life is about maintaining relationships with close others – whether friend or foe – and finding the space to identify the true nature of their thoughts and their feelings about them. And although she at first felt betrayed by her body turning against her, like Diski and Mayne, Taylor eventually accepts that even so, the cancer is part of her.

Gould and Hitchens believe their cancer to be a malignant alien; by temperament, they are outgoing and polemical rather than introspective and self-contained. For introverts Diski, Mayne and Taylor, however, who believe their cancer to be part of themselves, everything in their world – whether positive or negative – is experienced and scrutinised within, where they seek to investigate its nature, and understand its springs.

Is the cancer seen as part of the self? Summary

There are three different attitudes amongst the participants to the source of and thus, to their perspective on the cancer. Hitchens and Gould are engaged in a war to the death against an alien invader; accepting the notion of co-habitation with the cancer would be anathema to them. Mayne and Diski see the cancer as part of themselves; accordingly, they tolerate harbouring it, and reflect on how they can best relate to it. On this view, they can decide that undergoing the treatment damages their quality of life more than living with the cancer does, a position never adopted by Hitchens or Gould. Taylor believes that even if the cancer is part of her, it is antagonistic to her welfare. Accordingly, if this internal enemy goes too far and threatens to destroy her ability to live with herself, she reserves the right self-euthanise; that is, in effect, to save her intrinsic self by killing the internal saboteur. Possibly, an understanding of variations such as these in how the disease is perceived by cancer patients themselves, could be relevant to securing their commitment to a treatment regime; this is discussed further in Chapter 8, *Themes in the experience of dying.*

Does accepting cancer as part of the self lead to a 'better' death?

Do those who accept cancer as part of themselves also accept their dying and death without bitterness and therefore, have a 'better' death than those who do not? Is their death less distressed and more accepting because there is less balking at letting go? In this study, three participants believe that the cancer is part of the self – Mayne, Diski and Taylor – while the other two – Hitchens and Gould – see the cancer as an invader from without.

Once Mayne accepts that his death is near, he decides to reject further treatment in order to prioritise quality of life: "These last days [are about] … [the] quality, the living of this earthly life as fully as possible to the end" (Mayne, p. 246). Diski may or may not have decided to abandon the final round of chemotherapy; in any event, she cannot come to terms with approaching death, and remains troubled and unsettled until her memoir abruptly stops. Taylor's ten-year experience of increasingly symptomatic cancer has shown her that there is no way for her to escape death; without specifying what they are, she observes that once this fact has been understood, positive effects can result. Perhaps these 'positive effects' are not tangible but rather, relate to her finding that she can sustain her composure in the face of death's now imminent approach.

By contrast with these three participants, Gould and Hitchens continue to access every treatment possible to fight the cancer to the end, but when faced with it, like Mayne and Taylor, they accept that death is imminent without argument. As Gould sees it, it was only when he had accepted death that he felt free of its power and dominance, while Hitchens notes matter-of-factly that inevitably, he spends a good deal of time preparing himself to die.

There is, however, a practice common to them all, which does almost certainly play a positive role in how they work through the months, sometimes years-long period between diagnosis and death. This is not the first time that this activity has been observed and recorded, but in what follows, it is described and given a name.

Creative disregard

It would appear that regarding the cancer as part of the self is not a critical factor in readying oneself for death. However, there is some evidence that something else – the ability to put aside the preoccupation with illness and immerse oneself in a treasured project – might play a significant part in doing so. To achieve this, a degree of *creative disregard* must be undertaken; the individual must be able to emerge from the rage and pain of contracting a devastating illness, and re-invest in life beyond their own immediate health concerns. For example, for some years after the cancer diagnosis and the removal of her melanoma, Taylor had been well enough to work. She had published two long-postponed, highly praised novels before her death became imminent, followed by the memoir as her final publication. Hitchens continued his beloved lecturing and writing as much as his ill-health would allow. Gould returned to political campaigning while still well enough, and later completed a previously unfinished book about UK politics; he concluded his memoir literally on his deathbed. Mayne's memoir was combined with a substantial collection of final reflections on his theological insights. By contrast, Diski – hitherto a prolific and diverse writer – had no respite from the turbulence she endured from the diagnosis onwards; she was steadied by working on the memoir, but seemed to lack the resources to write anything else. Perhaps her description of her way of working best explains how her output became restricted to her own immediate concerns: "I'm a writer .... I write fiction and non-fiction, but it's almost always personal. I start with me, and often enough end with me" (Diski, pp. 10–11). Deprived of a flightpath to the future and unable to use her imagination to explore the world of otherness, Diski seems to have become caught in the confines of her own immediate present and its roots in the past.

Does accepting cancer as part of the self lead to a 'better' death? Summary

This study finds no confirmation for the hypothesis that accepting cancer as part of the self enables a 'better' death. However, one resource that the four participants who ultimately accepted death did have in common was the capacity for *creative disregard*, the ability to focus on a range of projects of general interest rather than solely on their own tribulations. Perhaps being able to come to terms with dying depends partly on having reached a stage of life at which preoccupation with the self has given way to an investment in others and otherness. If this is right, becoming aware of oneself as also being an other – a part of the sweep of history, and of the life cycle of the planet and its inhabitants – may represent an important stage in the process of letting one's own particular life go. Accordingly, creative disregard acknowledges the death sentence, but permits it to be put aside for the time being to allow for the commitment to some precious last contributions to the world of others – always provided, of course, that it is understood that when death finally approaches, it will be given its due. For individuals such as these participants, creative disregard comes naturally, but others may need encouragement to identify possibilities, and to invest in them; but there is no reason to suppose that for them, this would be less worthwhile than for those who needed no external guidance.

The second of three chapters of the participants' narrative, Chapter 6, *Living with dying*, follows the participants through the months they were to spend living and working while at the same time, their illness was progressing towards its terminal phase.

References

Anderson, S. (2017, November 29). *Euthanasia in Victoria: How the state's assisted dying laws will work* [ABC News]. Retrieved from http://www.abc.net.au/news/2017-11-22/euthanasia-in-victoria-how-assisted-dying -laws-will-work/9115210

Broom, A. (2012). On euthanasia, resistance and redemption: The moralities and politics of a hospice. *Qualitative Health Research*, *22*(2), 226–237. doi: 10.1177/104973231142181

Diski, J. (2016). *In gratitude*. London and New York: Bloomsbury Publishing.

Elias, N. (1985). *The loneliness of the dying*. E. Jephcott (Trans.). Oxford: Basil Blackwell Ltd.

Gould, P. (2013). *When I die: Lessons from the death zone*. London: Abacus, Little, Brown Book Group.

Health Research Funding. (2014, July 13). 25 surprising physician assisted suicide statistics. *Psychological Articles and Infographics*, Health Research Funding, 13/07/14. Retrieved from https://healthresearchfunding.org/physician-assisted-suicide-statistics/

Hitchens, C. E. (2012). *Mortality*. New York, Boston: Twelve Books.

Hutchinson, S. (2017, December 20). Living with a dying law. *The Australian, Weekend Inquirer*, p. 12.

Mayne, M. C. O. (2006). *The enduring melody*. London: Darton, Longman & Todd.

Murphy, B., & Ibrahim, J. (2018, March 6). Too many Australians living in nursing homes take their own lives. *The Conversation: Health and medicine*, p. 1. Retrieved from http://theconversation.com/too-many-australians-living-in-nursing-homes-take-their-own-lives-92112

Taylor, C. (2016). *Dying: A memoir*. Melbourne: Text Publishing.

Tucker, T. (2009). The culture of death denial: Relevant or rhetoric in medical education? *Journal of Palliative Medicine, 12*(12), 1105–1108. doi: 10.1089/jpm.2009.0234

Zimmermann, C. (2007). Death denial: Obstacle or instrument for palliative care? An analysis of clinical literature. *Sociology of Health and Illness, 29*(2), 297–314. doi: 10.1111/j.1467–9566.2007.00495.x

6 Living with dying

Introduction

As their illness progresses, the participants are confronted with an increasing number of issues on which they need to have a position, or make a decision. Death is still some way off and, as for all of us, is something of an abstract concept. However, the participants are by now deeply preoccupied with dying, and having the time to do so, they are struggling to understand what it means for them and in particular, how they can hope to die as safely and as peacefully as possible. The chapter which follows examines this aspect of their experience under two main headings – their attitudes towards dying, and how they go about preparing for it. As in the case of the previous chapter, Parts I and II of this investigation are further divided into a number of sub-sections.

Part I. Attitude to death and dying (*What the participant thinks death is; Attitude to death; Imagining dying; Attitude to dying*)

Part II. Preparation for and management of dying (*Planning for death; Considered Advance Care Planning; Considered voluntary euthanasia; Refused or sought life-prolonging treatment; Attitude to medical professionals; Meaningfulness in life and in dying*)

Part I. Attitude to death and dying (*What the participant thinks death is; Attitude to death; Imagining dying; Attitude to dying*)

What the participant thinks death is

As discussed in Chapter 2, *Death as enigma,* Part I, conceptualising one's own death is impossible and in fact, before receiving his terminal diagnosis, Mayne registers this: "Not that it is possible to imagine your own death" (Mayne, 2006, p. 92). Once in receipt of the diagnosis, however, and reflecting on what death means to him as a Christian, he can turn to the frame of reference held by the Anglican church: "In that ongoing relationship with our Creator... death is but the sloughing-off of the earthly body" (Mayne, p. 121) and, nearing the end of his life, when his religious beliefs are a prime

DOI: 10.4324/9781003392088-6

source of strength and consolation, he observes: "Our lives are sheer gift ... 'rounded with a sleep' as they transmute from one phase to the next ... is as natural as being born" (Mayne, p. 250). After receiving a terminal diagnosis and facing imminent death, Gould defines death experientially; he says that he is now living in the "Death Zone". Defining this as the time a dying person believes that they have left, Gould goes on to describe its strikingly contrasting landmarks: Acknowledging that death can leave you feeling somehow unfinished and that it is a sorrowful time, he says that for him, it is also a period of transformation, of transition and exhilaration. To explain her view of death, atheist Taylor resorts to evolutionary theory, defining death as a function of the need of all living things for a life cycle of death, revitalisation and renewal in the service of survival. Hitchens shows no interest in the subject.

Alone amongst the participants, Diski has reflected on the nature of death since she was a child: "Both infinity and death were beyond me .... [A]lthough I came to know that everyone was subject to death, it was some time before the penny dropped that I too would eventually be part of ... everyone who dies" (Diski, 2016, p. 141). In fact, Diski has struggled vainly to conceptualise personal death: "I vaguely grasped that the end of the infinite might be where death started" (p. 140). Once more the only participant to do so, she distinguishes between death and being dead; she understands the anxiety caused by not being able to capture and thus tame "death" or "being dead" with words:

> Death is the end of you. There is no being dead .... The horror of being unable to imagine it [is] ... because it is beyond the you that [can] ... think about it. I came up against the horizon of language.
>
> (p. 141)

She concludes: "[I'm] looking at death as negativity ... as absence" (pp. 143–144). She cannot take comfort from believing in an afterlife: "I'd never been envious of those who believe in an afterlife until now ... can't manage it" (pp. 157–158). But her death does become palpable to her when she identifies with her husband's sorrow: "When the Poet expresses his sadness and forthcoming grief, it hits me as if I were him suffering his loss of me .... a mirroring of another soul .... How else can I conceive of my own death?" (p. 142).

What the participant thinks death is: Discussion

None of the participants can conceptualise their own death; Mayne turns to his Christian beliefs about an afterlife, Taylor settles for an evolution-based view of death's function and Gould describes his experience of living in the Death Zone. After struggling with it for many years, Diski attributes her failure to conceptualise her death to the limits of language, though she can feel death's reality and power when she identifies with her husband's grief. On this subject, Hitchens makes no contribution.

Note that the special conditions required for a group of people to be able to talk about their own death is discussed in Chapter 2, *Death as Enigma,* Part II, where a community of elders living close to death developed an allusive private language to talk about it amongst themselves.

Attitude to death

Even though they cannot conceptualise their own death, once having been given a terminal diagnosis, all participants except Mayne have strong responses to it. In a formal response, Mayne quotes a fellow theologian: "'He who holds me in existence now ... will hold me in it still through and beyond the dissolution of my mortal frame'" (Mayne, p. 251). By contrast, the other participants have more personal views about death. Observing that it requires some resolution to study your own death, Taylor again refers to how lonely it is. As an atheist, she has no belief in an afterlife; her intuition is that we emerge from a void and that when we die, we are destined to return there. But she hopes for a different kind of immortality; now and then, she imagines that after she has died, somebody might pick up or browse a book of hers, and feel a moment of rapport with her as its author.

Now well past the initial diagnosis, Diski and Hitchens have both become more expressive about death as their constant companion. Dread of death lies in wait for Diski daily; she cannot put it aside and lose herself in ordinary life: "Death feels your collar when you're going about your business as if nothing has happened" (Diski, p. 143). Further, she cannot make her mind obey her veto on fearful brooding over it: "At least [I'm] ... not horrified with constant thoughts of death. I do think constantly of my death .... I watch and feel for symptoms .... So I think I'd better not be afraid, I'll always be afraid" (Diski, p. 243). Indeed, death's ominous presence has blocked out the light: "From being alive and making the human assumption that I will be around 'in the future', to coming to terms with a more imminent death. And then death itself. And there is no and" (Diski, p. 148). Hitchens visualises death as a lackey, given to loitering in wait in the passageways of his home. He is not particularly concerned about this creature's presence or even, about the knowing way it keeps handing him his coat; it is its perpetual sniggering that brings him undone. By now, his voice has been reduced by the treatment to an impotent squeak and his hands are losing the strength needed to type; he has lost faith in his robust intrepidity. Indeed, where once, in the words of the old saying, he would have declared: 'whatever doesn't kill me makes me stronger', he now asks himself why he ever thought it so full of wisdom.

Gould alone finds entering what he calls the Death Zone an absolute revelation, and he is on a mission to tell the world what he has discovered there. The number one item on his agenda has been to establish that as the cancer has returned, he has completely accepted that death is both real and imminent. Naturally, this process has taken time. When he first realised that death had finally gained the upper hand and that he was no longer in charge of his destiny, he had felt trapped in the inevitability of it all; death would trample him and his beloved family into the ground, and he would just have to submit to it. Having thus given his impending death due recognition, he recovers his usual sanguine outlook; he calls on us all to stand firm when facing death and, following his example, to look it straight in the eye. His prescription for survival in the Death Zone, this formula has never failed him.

Certainly, Gould does understand that death represents the troubling unknown; he recognises that there is a disconcerting new unpredictability in his own life, an ever-widening gap between the everyday world he knows so well, and whatever life after death is like. Nevertheless, he is not prepared to be intimidated; he realises that no one can defeat death, but he has found the courage to look it squarely in the eye, and refuse to blink. He makes us a promise; if someone says straight out to you that you are going to die, don't back away; instead, do what he does – look death right in the eye – and *at that very moment*, you will gain your freedom. And another thing: trying to duck the issue doesn't pay – if you keep saying 'yes, but *may*be this', or '*may*be that', you will be giving up on really living, on striving for freedom, and worst of all, on having a good death. Far from going downhill in that tragic way, Gould has found that death is a most fulfilling time for himself and for those close to him. In fact, he feels that the very intensity of death has given living a new power; he has had the opportunity to experience the most profound feelings, and to bring about reconciliations that would never otherwise have taken place. Finally, he has reached a state of complete openness and honesty with his wife, Gail, who fully reciprocates; he feels that their relationship has reached an intensity that they had never experienced before.

By this time, Gould has moved into a quasi-mystical state of mind; reflecting on the last five months, he can truly say that he has had more moments of sheer happiness, even of quiet ecstasy, than in the previous five years. Indeed, he feels completely at peace with the world. Now close to death, he is ready. Standing beside his recently chosen grave allotment in Highgate Cemetery, he finds himself thinking that he is deeply happy to be going to this place. And in these, his last days, his way of living has been transformed. Nowadays, he charts his course by the reference points of feelings and emotions, empathy and love.

For the first time in the investigation, the data obtained has covered the entire period from the initial diagnosis to the participants' final weeks of life, though with only a single entry, Mayne is so far reserved. Taylor remains steady and succinct, but feels the loneliness of dying; she dreams that she might be thought of in future by those who read her books. Hitchens reduces the Grim Reaper to a sniggering servant, but admits that the constant gloating presence finds its mark; he acknowledges that he is becoming weaker. Diski is beleaguered by thoughts of death; they catch her unawares, defy her vows not to be afraid, and remind her that she has no future. There is as yet no acceptance of death for Diski, and few moments of equanimity.

Gould advocates eyeballing death – especially when overtaken by fear – and aware that one cannot defeat or bargain with death, he intends to rise above it. Although a Christian believer in the afterlife, Gould believes that it is essentially because he has only a short time to live that his every moment has become intense and at times, ecstatic. Now, it might be wondered if Gould's accounts of such rapturous experience – unique among the participants – suggest that he has succumbed to some kind of quasi-delusional condition; perhaps he has lost control of the manipulation of all his emotions into positive channels and is now trapped on a perpetual high? On this view, Gould's demeanour and reports of his experience in his last weeks would sound grandiose and would not ring true. However, he does not advocate arrogantly vowing to defeat death but rather, suggests ways to face it squarely, and to rise above the fear it evokes. Arguably, this is not how someone in a persistently elevated mood would talk about meeting impending death; it sounds more like courage and imagination in adversity. If this is right, perhaps coming face-to-face with death can induce a profound psycho-spiritual experience in some people. Rather than an aberration, it may be for them, quite in character.

Attitude to death: Summary

As death approaches, the five participants experience it quite differently. Mayne is so far reserved, but he has more to say later. Taylor remains calm about accepting her death, but she feels lonely. Caring as her husband is, perhaps there is someone, a companion in facing death, for whom she seems to be searching. Hitchens is not afraid of death *per se* but he has acknowledged how vulnerable illness and the fear of an unmanageable death can make him feel. As her death approaches, Diski's lifelong use of her intellect and will to hold herself together as a coherent whole is beginning to break down; she finds herself unable to control or resolve her conflicted thoughts about her oncoming death. Gould finds that his perception of life as vibrant and absorbing is becoming ever more intense; now that death is upon him, his mood is bordering on the mystically ecstatic.

All of the participants have been much affected by the experience of having cancer and facing death; some are becoming stronger and more in charge of themselves and their destiny – for example, Christian believers, Mayne and Gould – or more complete, more able to acknowledge their fears and vulnerabilities – for example, Hitchens and Taylor. As death approaches, their enhanced awareness of what they are like, and what is important to them, has culminated in their becoming more fully themselves. Only Diski has stalled. She knows that she *will* die but unlike the other participants, she cannot find inscribed within herself the innate knowledge that she *can* die; something, somewhere in her past seems to have rendered it lost to her.

Imagining dying

As Mayne observes, being a believer does not free one from the fear of dying: "Our human fear of dying doesn't invalidate the Christian belief in resurrection ... fear of the dark and the unknown are common to us all" (Mayne, p. 92). However, what really concerns him in his weakened state is the possibility of losing touch with his faith, or with the capacity to think:

> [Remembering] ... the post-operative days when I was ... very scared .... Glimpsing what it might feel like to lose control of the power to think clearly or know that your faith is strong enough to face down your fears.
>
> (Mayne, p. 190)

For Gould, finishing his book on politics has brought with it a persistent sense that once he has completed the work currently in progress, his objective in life will be fulfilled, and the end will be in sight. If that is the case, in six weeks at the most, he will be dead. Moreover, from now on, he will have to confront more and more alarming symptoms every day. But whenever he feels his life racing to the finishing line like this, he knows what he must do; turn around, find the fear, and face it.

Confronted by moribund cancer patients in the radiotherapy waiting room, Diski is brought up sharply against the reality of death and dying:

> What was clear was the distinction between those of us who were having 'curative' radiotherapy and those of us who were not long for this world .... [Some] ... arrived in beds pushed by porters, all of them grey of face and still .... Others ... sat grimly with various wounds and scars from surgery, breathing heavily, [not] ... looking around at other patients waiting. We – the less ill ones – stole glances at these patients .... [We] ... must have seen the mirror the bedridden held up for us.
>
> (Diski, p. 131)

Even so, for Diski, the greatest torment still lies in what goes on in her head: "To be told that with an effort I might live for another two or three years brought back the uncertainty .... Can I learn to live with certain uncertainty, or uncertain certainty?" (Diski, pp. 138–139). Dying frightens her more than death: "Whatever terror there is lies in the present fear of dying, not so much of death" (Diski, p. 162), and: "I've got no apparatus to throw over myself as I make the swan dive. I'm just out there .... entirely alone" (Diski, p. 207); moreover: "I am scared of dissolution ... of knowing nothing when knowing everything has been the taste every day" (Diski, p. 244). Finally, while spending respite time in the local hospice, she is disturbed by hearing a woman moaning in unending misery: "'What is the matter with her?'.... The nurse ... said calmly, 'She's not ready. She hasn't thought enough about it and now it's very hard for her.' That's how I imagined dying .... I wanted help with that" (Diski, p. 212).

Imagining dying is one topic to which both Taylor and Hitchens also contribute freely. By now in her final year of eleven spent dying, Taylor finds that her mother's experience of dying from dementia in an institution remains imprinted on her memory. When she visited her spirited and adored mother and found her speechless, bereft of all bodily control, and with her eyes full of anguish as she endured being toileted and cleaned up in front of her daughter, Taylor was horrified and dismayed. Later, Taylor wondered if her mother had wanted her help to die, but at the time, she had simply hoped desperately that her mother would die naturally, and soon. In fact, it took her mother several months to die, but Taylor never visited her again. Now facing death herself, and consumed with feelings of guilt for abandoning her mother, Taylor is afraid that she has lost her mother's protective presence forever. In fact, even more than that, she seems to have become convinced that she deserves to be punished – perhaps by having to endure a horrible death just like her mother's, a death which would condemn her to die helpless, humiliated and abandoned. Little wonder that until the end, she feels the need to have a self-euthanising drug to hand.

After being diagnosed, Taylor had for some years been able to work; now, however, although she can write a memoir, she is too weak to construct and plan a novel. Reflecting on the years that she has spent dying, she attributes the long period of her increasing infirmity to our contemporary way of dying. Characterised as it is by worrying ambiguities and never-ending episodes of hope deferred, Taylor believes that it leaves patients and their families traumatised and despondent. Indeed, for Taylor herself, dying is the toughest assignment she has ever had to carry out, and she wishes that it was all over. Still haunted by the memory of her mother's death, she has obtained a drug online with which to euthanise herself if her dying becomes unbearable. Daydreaming about how it would be if she were to make use of the drug, she envisages kissing her loved ones goodbye, and with fear and suffering banished, falling asleep forever; thus, a harsh or bitter death would be replaced by a far gentler farewell. In comparison with what is known about the bleak reality of euthanasia – especially its distressing effects on any attendant family members – Taylor is certainly romanticising her own euthanasia scenario. In the real world, however, this daydream cannot make the prospect of her death any kinder; she acknowledges that the true reason for her reluctance to take her own life is that suicide is so dangerous. In fact, words fail her when she thinks of the fearful abyss that is death.

Unwontedly, Hitchens contributes the most entries to this section. He is oppressed by how the treatment has been depriving him of clarity of thought and now, by how dying is draining him of vitality and energy. Recently, he has undergone an experience at an airport of being unable to breathe; another such episode could be his last. His main vehicle of self-expression, his voice, has been replaced by a falsetto chirp, and his hands are becoming numb, scarcely capable of servicing his writing and thinking. In fact, with every day that passes, he loses more and more of his resources, leaving him with less and less bodily capital with which to face the next round of losses. In addition, any hospital procedures involving the use of water bring on memories of his panic-stricken state when – even though voluntarily – he was subjected to water-boarding. As if that were not enough, he remains afraid that the chemotherapy will affect his mind, rendering him prey to the fantasy that the medical personnel attending to him are actually sadistically torturing him, as a prelude to a horrific execution. By now, he has little respite from death's hovering presence. Even reading what is written about him is losing its once heady appeal – he can't help thinking that soon, such articles will just be part of the blurb in some posthumous write-up. Like Gould, he is experiencing a giddying feeling that he has been pitched forward in time, and is now hurtling down to the wire.

Treatment or torture?

While they are still well enough to be involved in anticipatory worrying, for every participant there are significant fears associated with the dying process. Only Taylor claims that she will simply be glad when her dying is over. Having had a premonition of death after finishing his last book, Gould acknowledges a fear of being struck down by catastrophic symptoms; however, as always, he intends to seek the fear out and stare it down. Mayne and Hitchens both express a continuing anxiety that their cancer drugs may undermine their mental functioning as death approaches; they have both had a glimpse of how it would be to die in hell. But Hitchens' fear that his 'chemobrain' will imagine that, rather than treatment, it is torture that is being inflicted on him, raises another, more general concern; how *do* we distinguish medical treatments from torture? Many treatments are painful or frightening but because our minds have normally learnt to distinguish medical treatment from abuse, we can instruct our bodies to endure it where possible.

Arguably, though, our distress tolerance will only hold if we are confident that we will be able to discriminate between medical care and torture. As is seen later in this chapter, Taylor worries about her Advance Care Plan's rejection of life-prolonging interventions at the end, exemplifying the anxiety that such ambiguities in the administration of Care plans can cause. Not sure if her decision to refuse nourishment involves medical support, she realises that if it should turn out that it does not, she has no idea how long it takes to starve to death, or if it is painful; even worse, she shudders at the thought of her adult sons seeing her die so tragically. Witnessing a loved mother's dying in torment is an image all too familiar to her.

The possibility of exposing the dying to intolerable pain or privation, and to experiencing their final days or hours as unintended torture, is discussed further in Part II of this chapter, in relation to treatment refusal in Advance Care Planning.

'Doing' dying

A second significant issue raised by the participants is their felt readiness to undergo the dying process. After hearing a dying woman moaning in anguish, Diski realises that she is equally unready to die, and that she needs counselling to help her to prepare herself. Dying is a universal experience, of course, and ordinarily, it begins as soon as the cues that govern the dying process are activated. For Diski, however, who seems to believe that it has only been learning what others know instinctively about how things work that has allowed her to be part of human society, knowing nothing about dying is especially confronting. Hence, she is desperate to find out in advance how dying is 'done'; if she remains uninitiated, she imagines that she will die, fully conscious and alone, abandoned to meltdown and dissolution. In Diski's system of 'Knowing everything is my all-time shield', such is the penalty for ignorance of something that in fact, before the event, nobody knows.

Actually, fearing dying more than death is not uncommon; according to Henry Fielding in *Amelia* (1751), "It hath been often said that it is not death, but dying, which is terrible."

In Diski's nightmare scenario, we may not know how to 'do' dying, but we will just have to go ahead anyway, and be mangled by it. And yet, dying is one of those events in life about which, typically, we have no choice and play no initiating part; it is inscribed in our psyche in the same way as being born is. It seems probable that on the day, all we can, or need to do, is to go with the flow. If this is right, the main difficulty for Diski – and perhaps for those who share her anxiety – is that not being in control at all times is unendurable. With death on the horizon, Diski finds that she cannot bypass the inscription – perhaps something like "Play possum, but *never surrender*" – which, during her oft-beleaguered lifetime, has overwritten everything else in her psyche, including the unconscious knowledge that dying takes care of itself. And although Diski's is a defining case, arguably, the "Dying happens naturally" inscription is generally becoming harder to access in a society as death-avoidant as ours; we need to take care that it does not become extinct.

None of the other participants expresses an inability to imagine themselves dying, although they frequently allude to the fear and sadness it involves. This matter is further discussed later in this chapter, and in the next, and last, data analysis narrative chapter.

Imagining dying: Summary

All the participants have their own fears about dying; some of these are shared with one or more others. Mayne, Gould, Taylor and Diski all find that dying is intrinsically frightening because it is unknown territory and so final, but they deal with their fear in different ways. Mayne and Taylor accept and allow their anxiety to pass, while Gould stares his anxiety down, but Diski has no such recourse; she seeks counselling because she has a persistent fear that she cannot 'do' dying.. Hitchens does not express fear of dying *per se*, but worries that in his drugged state, it could masquerade as torture and murder.

Taylor and Diski are both finding the lengthy dying period hard to endure and the uncertainty of how events will progress disturbing; Taylor is concerned about what families have to endure, while Diski feels haunted by moving closer to dying while still unready for it. By now close to death, Hitchens and Gould both report that, on occasion, they have a vertiginous sense of being rushed to the finishing line.

Attitude to dying

Mayne makes no contributions to this sub-category as yet. All the other participants have by now entered the final straight; their earlier, wider-ranging commentary has become focused on their individual narratives about the experience of dying.

Now weeks from death, Gould advises the inhabitants of the Death Zone to live life to the full. In aid of this, they should get rid of pain by any means possible, so as to have as many quality days as they can. Well aware that he will have to endure some harrowing periods with the fulminating cancer in his stomach before he dies – the worst of times – he also has days that he regards as by far the best times of his life. A standout for his continuing upbeat approach to his death, Gould is also remarkable for his capacity to hold ordinarily opposed states of body and mind together in his consciousness – for example, Death Zone/best quality days, and worst of times/best of times. By contrast, Hitchens concentrates on trying to rid himself of attitudes which he now regards as ambivalent, negative or weak, retaining only those which he finds straightforward and deserving of his approval. He has already determined to shut down becoming self-absorbed and sorry for himself, and from now on, he has no intention of allowing an anxious preoccupation with the ups and downs of the tumour to dominate his thoughts. Indeed, as it turns out, although they are so different in attitudes and temperament, Hitchens and Gould are alike in one central respect; in spite of the temptation to give way to fear or self-pity as they face terminal illness and death, both men vow to remain undaunted by it. In short, come what may, they will not be bullied by the enemy alien, the cancer; they intend to remain themselves, writ large.

Having had so many years to reflect on it, Taylor has contributed more entries to how she sees dying than any other participant; as many sociologists have done before her, Taylor has also mulled over the secularisation of our society, and how it has left us without common rituals or language with which to relate to dying. As an atheist, she feels conflicted about turning to frameworks which rely on our still being connected to our religious heritage, but on the other hand, she feels lost in the face of having to extemporise, to create her own *ars moriendi*. Another aspect of dying that she finds challenging, is having to live in a dying body which no longer feels like an integral part of herself. As someone who had enjoyed being at one with the pleasures of her body from childhood, she was shocked by the physical damage caused by the cancer and its treatment over the years. And now that her body is so unsightly and disfigured, she feels cut off from it; all she wants to do is to put it aside. Now become an inscrutable other, however, this body has its own program for meeting death. In fact, given that she is doing it for the first time, Taylor finds that much of dying remains a mystery to her; thinking about it can still make her momentarily anxious, but unlike Diski, for Taylor, the uneasiness soon passes. At the same time, what she does know by now is that there are good things associated with dying slowly in the way that she is. Perhaps best of all, she has had time to let people know how much she cares for them, and to try to make sense of the life that is ending; looking back over it, she realises how restorative it has been to remember the things that she has done, and to resist hankering after those that she has not.

In complete contrast, for Diski, there is no relief from fear and anxiety:

> The excruciating terror ... of dying comes regularly and settles on my solar plexus directly beneath my ribcage .... There the terror squats, rat or raptor, its razor-sharp claws digging into that interior organ where all dreaded things ... live in me.
>
> (Diski, p. 143)

She has been offered one last drug trial which might briefly lengthen her life, but it has little appeal: "I don't exactly feel ill now. I'm trapped in a mesh of steroid effects .... Fat that feels like my body has been stuffed with some alien gel .... It's like a punishment. But for what?" (Diski, p. 208). It is of interest to note here that according to Kubler-Ross, everyone experiences death as a punishment, but Diski is actually the only participant to do so; note, too, that she is still in a state of radical disbelief, experiencing the treatment, and not the cancer, as the source of the feeling that she is being punished. At this stage feeling close to death, she has begun taking the latest round of drugs: "I'm very feeble but .... here I am, thinking and taking pills, wondering whether the fibrosis will kill me first or the tumour .... It was Christmas, and probably my last" (Diski, pp. 244–245). Being in terror of dying has not led Diski to retreat into denial; always watchful and alert in a world which never feels secure, she remains painfully aware of her condition.

Sometime before Diski became ill, her daughter, Chloe, had a son, and two years later, quite recently, a daughter. As the loss forever of these small grandchildren draws closer, Diski mourns the separation from them in a heartfelt way that she seldom allows herself to express: "Meantime ... there's the two-year-old grandson .... I'll be in some books and photographs and a few stories he's been told .... That's what really distresses me" (Diski, p. 155); "I feel the sadness even more sharply, now that the new girl child has been born, at the idea of missing knowing what they will both be like" (Diski, p. 156), and: "The loss of the future children and grandchildren is unbearable, although ... quite in the way of things .... the insoluble grief" (Diski, p. 239). In despair, however, she does not believe that this dawning capacity for unconditional love can help to shepherd her through dying:

> There's only one piece of magic left if faith is left out. Love, there's love. But if I arrived on earth without a capacity for faith ... with a death sentence tattooed on me ... how the hell am I going to place my trust in love?
> (Diski, p. 207)

Attitude to dying: Summary

In different ways, three of the participants are by now composing themselves for dying. Gould embraces all of his qualities – whether inconsistent or even opposites – while now that he is dying, Hitchens vows not to indulge those weaknesses brought on by the illness. Both intend to die as they have lived, writ large. After ten years of illness, Taylor has little fear of dying, and has found reflecting on what she has done rather than hankering after what she has not, gives her solace. Diski remains fearful, angry and despairing; she is well aware that she will soon die, but she cannot accept it. Having recently received a terminal diagnosis, the fifth participant, Mayne, has yet to respond.

Part II. Preparation for and management of dying

(Planning for death; Considered advance care planning; Considered voluntary euthanasia; Refused or sought life – prolonging treatment; Attitude to medical professionals; Meaningfulness in life and in dying)

Now in their last months, the participants are addressing two matters which are of the first importance to them. Firstly, now that death is imminent, they reflect on what has mattered most to them in life, and secondly, having decided on the kind of death they hope to have, they must make decisions about trying to ensure it. Part of their preparation involves practical arrangements like planning a funeral or making an Advance Care Plan; this is explored in the present chapter. The more intangible aspect of making ready – of meeting death with acceptance – is explored in the next and final chapter of this participant narrative.

Planning for death

Written when she is nearing death, Diski's entries about her prospective funeral are as always, subversive of customary social rituals. Discussing her prospective death with her husband, she wants him to lighten up: "I don't much care about the funeral arrangements, but if I'm going to be buried, I want to be tucked up in a winter tog-rated duvet" (Diski, p. 142). Her other comment addresses the reader, and is typically satirical: "I don't think I want a funeral. Very last year .... Always fancied '*Smoke Gets in Your Eyes*' and for the Poet to sing a properly political song .... Also ... the *Grosse Fuge*" (Diski, pp. 245–246).

By contrast, in their different ways, Gould, Hitchens, Mayne and Taylor do attend to the duties dying imposes on them. Before his first surgery – when he still expects a cure – Gould nevertheless makes a will and organises his funeral. In the event of his possibly not surviving the surgery, he writes a farewell letter to every member of his family, breaking down completely as he writes. Although like Gould, still hopeful of a cure, Mayne also plans his funeral before his first surgery: "Type out ... details of choice of funeral service. Should have done it years ago" (Mayne, p. 46), and like Gould, he writes letters to his family members: "Write and file hasty but heartfelt letters to A., Mark and Sarah, 'just in case'" (Mayne, p. 49). Hitchens is typically matter-of-fact, merely noting that he has to spend time ensuring that his loved ones will be properly looked after.

With a terminal diagnosis in place and some months left to live, Taylor is practical and business-like. Finding it supportive both for them and for herself, she takes her family through the relevant paperwork, and shows them what she needs them to do. Having put some thought into her funeral, she feels the need for an element of sacred ritual and accordingly, she decides to ask a Buddhist nun she knows to say a prayer for her from the Tibetan Book of the Dead. By contrast, she puts rather less thought into the disposal of her remains; she decides to ask her husband, a ceramic artist with a studio in Japan, to decorate an urn for her ashes and then, to keep it with him until he is ready to toss her out. Taylor's attitude towards herself and her husband is puzzling here. From having addressed the funeral details up to that point with appropriate decorum, at the mention of her ashes being given to Shin as her next of kin, she breaks into rough, childish speech, referring to his having to "toss me out". As will also be seen in the next chapter, Taylor has a tendency to break into a similarly harsh way of talking when the conversation becomes distressing; as if in tacit rectification, this is often followed quite soon by a more mature and caring observation. In this case, the correction is swift, and comes as an expression of her concern for her husband and sons when they face the ritual of spreading her ashes; she realises that it will be difficult for them, and hopes that they will be a comfort to each other. At times like this, Taylor gives the impression that there are two unconnected inner voices operating independently within her, and that their communications to the world have not yet been harmonised into a more centralised, better integrated way of thinking and speaking. Perhaps the most glaring example of it to date occurred when, in contrast with her loving references to missing Shin and her sons, she seems not to realise what impact her confidences to her memoir about her intention to self-euthanise is likely to have on them. What this state of internal disunion might indicate, and how it finally works out for Taylor, is discussed in the next and last, participants' narrative chapter, *Acceptance*.

Planning for death: Summary

Mayne, Gould, and Taylor organise their affairs and their funerals with their families; Mayne and Gould write possibly last letters to their families prior to their first surgery, and with Hitchens, make provision for loved ones. Diski cannot make any genuine preparations. As a rule, people who are aware that they are dying need the opportunity to plan how they want to die; some creative *Ars Moriendi* scenarios are discussed in Chapter 8, *Themes in the experience of dying*.

Considered voluntary euthanasia

Taylor is the only participant to have considered voluntary euthanasia.

She first heard about Exit International and the debate around assisted dying from her mother, who had joined Exit long before either of them ever became ill. Sometime later, and faced with imminent death herself, Taylor intends to take control of her own death, in the way that she imagines her mother would have wanted her to do. Accordingly, she has already joined Exit International and now, as it becomes clear to her from her clinical test results that she will not live far beyond her sixtieth birthday, her thinking becomes concentrated on obtaining the means to die by voluntary euthanasia. She gives her reasons for this in her memoir – though still, not to her family – describing how fearful she is of having a 'bad death', in particular, by being trapped in agonising overtreatment by some medical professional who is refusing to let her go. When she does finally try to take her family into her confidence by telling them that, because she needs to have the means to take charge of how she is going to die – even if she never uses it – she is exploring medications suitable for use in self-administered euthanasia, she reports that they made no response. Curiously, she takes the family's silence to mean that they at least had no objection to her tentative plan; it did not seem to occur to her that her family may well have been so shocked and nonplussed by her declaration that they were lost for words. It is also possible that, if they were accustomed to some degree of eccentricity in Taylor's views – perhaps more so since she had become ill – their tacitly understood way of handling these moments was just to let them pass.

Eventually, Taylor does come to realise that she cannot expect her husband and sons to be involved in her euthanasia. Apparently unaware that their reluctance to participate in her suicide would have had its origin in the bonds of protective attachment between husband and wife, and parents and children, she does feel disappointed and angry about it. Rather than directing her displeasure at her family, however, she displaces it on to the pious, railing against them for obstructing the legalisation of euthanasia; she is convinced their God sets a high value on seeing people suffer. Having perhaps realised that the subject of her quest for euthanasia was too hot for her family to handle, she seems from then on to have saved her confidences about it for her memoir. On the other hand, she does feel free to exercise her capacity for trenchant comment on the management of her death with her GP; she reports that when he mentioned that for religious people, death can be more arduous because they believe that pain has a purpose, she informed her GP crisply that she would be fine with taking any painkillers she could get her hands on.

Having finally concluded that, apart from her friends at Exit International, she would probably have to manage her dying alone, Taylor found the means; two years previously, she had obtained a euthanasia drug from China. Worried that she might be disabled by the then proposed brain surgery, she welcomed the drug's arrival just a few days beforehand; together with a suicide note which she had written to her family before the brain surgery, she kept it in a private cache for use in the event of any subsequent emergency. In the suicide note she asks for forgiveness, explaining to her family that she has promised herself that if she came round from the surgery disabled and totally dependent, she would rather terminate her life. Then, after telling them how much she loved them, she ends the note with her heartfelt thanks for the pleasure and happiness that they have brought her. In fact, the note was never delivered; with some loss of function, Taylor survived the operation in better shape than she had feared. However, the success of the brain surgery did not alter her need to control how she would die; still imagining herself as a possible victim of a slow and hideous death, she felt that the drug offered her a kinder and more speedy passing which, above all, she could count on. Thinking about this as she writes, she pictures the scene: all of her family and special friends would be invited to say goodbye to her; first, she would declare her love for them and thank them for all that they had done for her, and then, farewell them, take the medication, and drift into eternal sleep. Convinced that nothing could be better than this vision for how her life should end, Taylor seems unaware that, from the point of view of the others involved, this scenario might appear distressing, even bizarre, and certainly something that they might very well not want to take part in.

This ability to drift to faraway shores when under stress comes from Taylor's creative imagination; at any time, she can construct and disappear into a world which for a time, is more vivid to her than everyday reality. While she is there, the characters she creates – often from people she knows intimately in life – can be made to do and say whatever her current scenario prescribes. But when she realises that her dream cannot be transformed into reality – in this case, that the beautiful death she pictures may never happen – her disappointment turns to anger. As she had blamed religious believers rather than her unresponsive family for dragging their feet over her plan to self-euthanise, she now blames Australian law prohibiting legally-assisted dying for turning what should be a sublime farewell into a serious crime. Now, it may be thought that Taylor had no regard for the law or for the feelings of others, but this is not so; at this point, having thus given herself an unwelcome wake-up call, her responsibilities in the real world flood back. First in line is her realisation that, given that she would never want to implicate anyone else in her suicide, she would have to die alone. Picturing this as a lone and tragic act rather than the wonderful farewell scenario of her dreams, she is horrified to think of the impact that killing herself would have on her husband and sons. On the other hand, the fear of becoming helpless and abandoned remains; she continues to argue that saving herself from such a fate should not be considered a criminal act. Accordingly, she cannot willingly discard the drug.

But then, suddenly, in the midst of this debate with herself, Taylor has a moment of truth: she wonders if it is because it is so very perilous that she is hesitant about killing herself. From then on, although she continues to mention it, the likelihood that she would ever actually make use of the drug seems to fade into obscurity.

Considered voluntary euthanasia: Summary

Taylor has revealed that the feared catastrophe of "dying badly" is, in fact, a fear of being immobilised by helplessness and becoming totally dependent on others – the fate which she believes to have overtaken her mother; it is to prevent anxiety about this possibility from overwhelming her that she retains the drug, but she is ambivalent about actually taking it. On the one hand, to be ready to activate her plan while she still has the capacity to do it, she has to keep the drug close by her; on the other, she is too frightened of committing suicide to make use of it. Her two 'voices' within – emanating from sets of images, whether fantasy or real world-based – continue to exist as alternating and opposed views which she can neither reconcile, nor encapsulate in an overarching third idea. For example, instead of being locked into whether or not to suicide, she could in theory make a sideways move and research care for the helpless dying – possibly in a hospice – and enlist her GP's help in establishing a link with it in preparation for her time of need; but at this stage, she seems reluctant to ask for help. Unable to work through her dilemma, she leaves it in the air; it will become increasingly apparent that, even when her failure to resolve a major issue runs counter to her declared intentions, Taylor is inclined to abandon the whole conflict and drift away. Arguably, the sapping of will brought about by her irresolution reveals an intuition that she might become helpless not as a hazard for the future, but rather, as one which, mentally rather more than physically, is already overtaking her.

A discussion of the many issues surrounding legally-assisted dying is outside the scope of this study, but it is noted that it has now been introduced in various countries, including in Australia; it became law first in Victoria, and more recently, in Western Australia, Tasmania, South Australia, Queensland and finally, in New South Wales. Since she did not suffer from severe and intractable pain, however, even if the legislation had been in place in her time, Taylor would not have qualified for legally-assisted dying, despite being terminally ill. Her concerns were about quality of life; for some commentators, the failure of the legislation to make provision for terminally ill people experiencing a poor quality of life, is a significant deficiency in the service that it is intended to provide.

Considered advance care planning

Only the women, Diski and Taylor, made Advance Care Plans.

Taylor's Plan is an extension of her euthanasia strategy; it is a directive to her palliative care specialist that because she wants nothing to impede the natural process of dying, she wants no life-prolonging treatment at the last. Diski's Plan has a different purpose; it is intended to avoid death through suffocation and just as importantly, the fear of it, by ensuring appropriate palliative care: "I still tell the doctor and hospice nurse both conversationally and in a signed living will that I want to die easily, not an agitated death" (Diski, p. 209).

None of the other participants made Advance Care Plans. The reasons Taylor and Diski give for doing so were for Diski, wanting to secure as easeful a death as possible, and for Taylor, to ensure that her death would not be delayed by last-minute attempts at treatment; these are two of the main objectives that Advance Care Planning aims to deliver. But for both Taylor and Diski, complications develop which could render their Plans futile; Diski's chosen hospice is unable to guarantee that the palliative care essential to the fulfilment of her Plan will be available, and as is seen in *Refused or sought life-prolonging treatment* immediately below, Taylor acknowledges having grave concerns about possible adverse effects on herself and her family if her Care Plan ever had to be activated.

Considered advance care planning: Summary

Only the two women participants made Advance Care Plans; the defining factor for both of them appears to be their uncertainty that they can rely on appropriate medical care being put in place when they are dying. However, there can be latent ambiguities inherent in Advance Care Plans which would need to be addressed if a Plan is to provide medical personnel with an accurate reading of its author's intentions.

Refused or sought life-prolonging treatment

With death approaching, all participants were faced with making decisions about whether to accept further harsh treatment in return for more time, or to reject it in favour of preserving a better quality of life.

Diski does not proactively seek either to access or to refuse treatment; rather, she is the passive recipient of proffered medication which she weighs up whether or not to accept: "A decline caused by fibrosis or lung cancer is very unpleasant. But … the prospect of stronger and nastier medication, left me thinking about the balance .... [Q]uality of life .... Versus, I suppose, no life at all" (Diski, pp. 160–161). She accepts a new and final trial medication: "I've been given one last chance. A trial pill .... The last lot I stopped because they made me sick ... These new ones have bad side-effects after which there is 'nothing we can do for you'" (Diski, p. 245). Persistent vomiting had made Diski stop chemotherapy before; it seems unlikely that she would make substantial use of this final offer. Mayne is faced with a similar dilemma; after suffering much brutal treatment and now in receipt of a terminal diagnosis, he has been offered a final round of chemotherapy. He does not hesitate: "I have said 'no' to aggressive chemotherapy. That leaves the possibility of a milder form .... but I know already what we'll opt for. Quality, not quantity of days" (Mayne, p. 250).

With cherished projects to complete, Gould and Hitchens have both always wanted more life. When his cancer recurred some time ago, Gould had been offered a second radical surgery. At first, he was unenthusiastic, but when he had asked how long he would live without the surgery, he was told that it would only be six months to a year. Reluctantly, he had agreed to the surgery, and although the cancer did recur, he secured the time he needed to complete his memoir and his book on politics. For his part, although his treatment has been very harsh, Hitchens has no complaints; on balance, he values the life it has given him. Reflecting on the issue of whether he would have opted for the treatment if he had known what it would be like, he does wonder at times. On the other hand, looking back, he acknowledges that really, there was never any question about it; if he had not had the treatment, he would be dead long since, and that does not interest him at all.

Again, Taylor is gripped by mutually incompatible pressures – this time, regarding life-prolonging treatment – and again, she cannot resolve her strong but opposed views. On the one hand, she remains committed to the wishes stated in her Advance Care Plan; firstly, she wants to keep open the possibility of a relatively quick death from pneumonia by refusing all antibiotics, and secondly, having also refused artificial nourishment, she is prepared, if necessary, to allow herself to die of starvation. On the other hand, however, she shudders at the thought of her sons being perpetually haunted by the memory of their mother looking like a concentration camp victim, and does not dare even to think about how it would affect her husband. As with the euthanasia issue, there is no resolution to this conflict. Given that she seems so determined to control the way she dies, Taylor is surprisingly neglectful about finalising conflicts which, if unresolved, may not only cause anguish for everyone but also, negate her intention to die easily and without hindrance. As with the euthanasia plan and the disposal of her ashes, Taylor first makes an emphatic statement in her Advance Care Plan, then expresses grave reservations about it and finally, lets the matter lapse unresolved. If her brain surgery might have affected her ability to make the kind of connections we need to make if we are to recognise antitheses and to bring them together to give rise to a new idea, Taylor seems to be unaware of it.

Refused or sought life-prolonging treatment: Summary

Whenever a participant is offered a late life-prolonging treatment, it is just that – a way to prolong life, not to enhance it. Hitchens and Gould accept all treatment proffered in order to have more time to work on their projects; Diski vacillates, but with no special projects to complete, she seems likely to reject a final round of treatment offering more life because it makes her so sick, while Mayne unhesitatingly rejects treatment to prolong life, in favour of retaining its quality. Taylor fails to resolve the question of whether her refusal of life-prolonging treatment at the end of life will be the way to a 'good' death, or render it hideous for all concerned. That she is persistently in two minds is examined further in Chapter 7 below, *Acceptance*.

In all, three participants – Diski, Mayne and Taylor – are concerned about the ill-effects of treatment, with two or perhaps all three deciding that more life would not be worth the loss of its quality, while two others – Hitchens and Gould – accept all treatments that offered them more time, in order to complete cherished projects; Diski does not record making a final decision. In general, the decision to seek or reject life-prolonging treatment varies according to the individual's lived experience of balancing tolerance of the suffering caused by the treatment against the desire for more life. Therefore, this study finds that while a desire to receive all available life-prolonging measures to the end does regularly occur, it is by no means universal amongst the dying.

Attitude to doctors and medical professionals

Hitchens, Gould and Mayne are mainly positive about their medical professionals, while Diski and Taylor are mainly negative about them.

Hitchens regards his doctors as top-notch allies in the fight for his life. In the opposite corner crouches the unseeing, coldly calculating alien, out to destroy him, but in his corner, committed to his ongoing living, there is a virtuoso team of specialists, all single-mindedly devoted to his care. Indeed, though normally reticent about his illness, Hitchens does sometimes respond when the staff at his cancer clinic ask after him; in a typically gnomic reply, he usually tells them that today, it would appear that he has cancer. Gould's experience of oncology consultants is more mixed. On the one hand, when reluctantly considering his second round of surgery, he reports how uplifted he felt when his second oncologist, David Cunningham, told him that he would fight alongside him all the way. On the other hand, he is less happy with the initial phase of his treatment; this is due mainly to a mistake he made at the outset when, underestimating the seriousness of his condition, he chose a less invasive surgery over the more radical proposal that he really needed to eradicate the cancer. When, later on, the cancer recurred and became terminal, he had to acknowledge that he had made a grievously wrong decision. In fact, at this point, he believes that his impending death may even be premature, the result of human error.

Unlike Hitchens and Gould, Mayne feels no need to research the field for the best advice; he accepts a referral to a local oncologist, the first specialist he sees: "I warmed to him at once" (Mayne, p. 45). Even after a first traumatic surgery, which took ten hours, and was followed by inadequate pain control and drug-induced nightmares, Mayne remains full of praise: "I also have a new admiration for the sheer professionalism of the cancer care team" (Mayne, pp. 77–78). Indeed, it is not until he has had damaging, and possibly unnecessary radiotherapy to his surgically-wrecked mouth – in an effort to eradicate some previously overlooked cancers – that his attitude changes: "'No one can be trusted.' Realise that throughout I have put my entire trust in the doctors .... Haven't questioned their judgment" (Mayne, pp. 218–219). Having soon afterwards received his terminal diagnosis, Mayne's praise of medical professionals becomes more selective: "I have grown in admiration for the skill and dedication of the best of the medical profession" (Mayne, p. 245). Indeed, despite its being suggested by his doctors, Mayne's decision to reject a final round of treatment illustrates how reliant on his own judgment he has finally become.

By contrast, both Diski and Taylor are generally dissatisfied with the medical professionals they encounter, though in Diski's case, there is a telling exception. Taylor's entries are all negative; having said that she has no wish to denigrate her doctors, she feels that she must nonetheless point out that only the palliative care specialists ever spoke to her about death. Actually, she did not even feel regarded as a person in her consultations with doctors; she would emerge feeling that her whole being had been diminished to a set of symptoms. Deciding to invest in seeing a specialist in death counselling, she had left the psychologist's office afterwards full of scorn, declaring that although the woman was obviously a well-educated whizz kid, all she had to offer were techniques of chilling out that anyone could get from Dr Google. In fact, she was obliged to report that no medical professionals had felt the need to address her dying, or for that matter, any other important personal issues with her.

Diski has similar complaints: "Everything is presented to me statistically, as probabilities. I can't find the right question to ... talk about the cancer that is me and mine" (Diski, p. 117), and in the context of radiation therapy:

> As soon as I was lying down ... one of the radiographers ripped ...apart [the smock] ... to reveal my naked upper torso .... A leaflet about the treatment ... [said] that my dignity was important .... My dignity was left at the door.
>
> (Diski, p. 123)

Her grievances resemble Taylor's; nobody in these encounters shows any concern for her as a person and moreover, they even seem indifferent to her well-being; during one of her radiation sessions: "Twice [the radiation machine] stopped ... I was eventually told ... that something had gone wrong with the computer .... I rather hoped that the computer [was not] ... aiming the wrong beams at the wrong place in me" (Diski, p. 126). Finally, in despair of ever experiencing any honest concern about her condition, she concludes: "I don't trust anyone" (Diski, p. 207).

It may sound as if Diski is indulging in a cynical beat-up when she says: "What could anyone give me that could definitively improve my health? .... when most of the unwellnesss came from the treatment?" (Diski, p. 207). However, what she says is true – at a certain point, cancer treatment can cause more suffering than the disease; she has become too fatigued to stay awake for more than a few hours a day, vomits on the pills, frequently fractures bones, and has regular bouts of near-suffocation because the radiotherapy for the tumour has also rendered her pulmonary fibrosis terminal. Still shuddering at the memory of an outburst from an overwhelmed GP, she is well aware that her prospects are grim: "[I am] ... haunted by the memory of my former GP saying .... 'Oh Jenny, they're both such terrible ways to die'" (Diski, p. 166). But there was one exception to Diski's experience of the general lack of concern for her welfare; her first, very attentive chemotherapy unit nurse, L., had gained Diski's confidence. Once the infusions were completed, however, Diski made a painful discovery: "As soon as I arrived at the oncology ward for the final infusion, I found myself ... distressed .... that 'my' designated nurse, L, would no longer be available to be called ... with 'any little problem'" (Diski, p. 118). As she left the ward for the last time, she was in tears; despite its distressing side effects, Diski had managed to accept a full round of chemotherapy when a policy of unconditional concern for every patient was in place.

Gender-based differences appear to exist in the participants' attitudes to the medical personnel they encountered. Even though they all endured harsh procedures, Mayne, Hitchens and Gould seem predominantly satisfied with the support and medical care they received; none of them complained about being treated without interest or concern as Taylor and Diski had done. It is possible that because all three of the male participants were well-known public figures, of whom two were titled, they might have attracted especially attentive treatment. Further, Gould and Hitchens were treated in highly-regarded private hospitals. In general, however, given that in our society men are expected to maintain their composure through pain and suffering, perhaps it suits them best if the delivery of their medical care is professional and efficient, rather than related and sympathetic.

But there is another aspect of the gender difference. From the outset, Diski and Taylor expect to have a relationship with their treating professionals which, even though they may develop a working alliance with certain of their doctors, the men do not appear to do. As often happens, most of the senior medical professionals involved with the participants were men. Now, if in the emotionally-charged context of serious illness settings, women in our society typically construe the contacts they have with medical staff in relationship terms, the mismatch between their expectations and those of most of their treating professionals will persist. Both Diski and Taylor felt diminished by it; any consequent lack of trust will cause distress to the patient, and may even compromise their capacity for compliance with treatment.

Attitudes to doctors and health professionals: Summary

Although generalisations cannot be made from such a small sample, it is possible that there are significant differences in the way that seriously ill men and women in our society react to the medical professionals that they encounter. Arguably, perhaps due to the expectations of them in our Western culture, men learn to distance themselves emotionally from suffering and damage. For women, however, when gravely ill, impersonal or distant treatment by health-care workers may be experienced as threatening to their already strained sense of self-identity; if so, this would lead them to seek – but perhaps not to find – more supportive relationships with their medical professionals. In an ideal world, the policy of unconditional concern that was on offer in Diski's first chemotherapy unit would represent the gold standard for supportive patient care. Given that none of the other participants mentioned having such an experience, however, it may be quite rare; perhaps new projects and a new kind of leadership is needed in the field of doctor-patient relationships.

Meaningfulness in life and in dying

Diski

With the smallest number of entries in this category, Diski's record of what is most meaningful to her is nonetheless eloquent. Firstly, she records what has provided her with a path to maturity and, given her suicidal youth, perhaps to survival itself: "'What's the point?' Only earning my living writing" (Diski, p. 213), extended in:

> The only answer to the miserableness of most of my childhood was that I ought to be a writer .... I'd wanted to be ... a journalist .... Later ... I realised that novelists lived exactly as I wanted to live.
>
> (Diski, p. 214)

Secondly, she expresses sorrow at the impending loss of her grandchildren: "I only feel deprived of not watching the grandchildren ... become their own people. For now, they remain delightful, a special medicine whose main side-effect is a painful sadness" (Diski, p. 211). Her grandson has taught her how, if loved, even small children can stand up to adult expectations: "My two-year old grandson, when asked a question he can't or doesn't want to answer, says after a moment: 'Ella' .... [Diski's ellipsis points]. I might adopt this ploy" (Diski, pp. 164–165). Seeing how children's play can give them a sense of mastery – the obverse of her own experience – in her imagination, she uses it to parody "Onc Doc": "'There's nothing else we can do for you.'

Doc language for 'You've failed us and you'll just have to die, which is not our speciality, so goodbye.' Or as my grandson would put it, 'Ella'" (Diski, p. 167). Again, she mourns: "The ...loss ... of the future children and grandchildren is unbearable .... The insoluble grief" (Diski, p. 239). Trapped in her inimical inner world, this glimpse of the world of a loved toddler – sprung from her own flesh and blood – seems to have allowed her an at once first, and final, bittersweet glimpse of how a child can grow up in a secure and loving world.

Being always creatively engaged in the writing life as she has been for thirty years is no longer an option for Diski; exhausted and weak, and lacking a sense of future, or of relatedness to anything beyond her own dark world, she has lost the motivation to write anything other than her memoir. However, she does feel a unique tenderness towards her grandchildren, and experiences a painful joy whenever they come to visit. Indeed, despite her perception of herself as beyond the reach of love, she seems to grieve over the impending loss of these loved ones as deeply as the other participants grieve over theirs. Perhaps the saddest irony of Diski's life is not her terror of death but rather, that she has such a short time to enjoy, and even be mended a little, by the gift of unconditionally loving her grandchildren.

Gould

According to Gould, much has been gained from reviewing his experience of having cancer and more recently, of facing death. Being close to death and undergoing severe pain has made him better able to tolerate these ordeals, but also, more empathic, and thus, more compassionate towards other sufferers. The cancer experience has also led him to review his commitment to the Anglican faith; having found that it had failed to sustain him *in extremis*, he can see that his faith has become more questioning and less naively trusting – actually, more congruent with his personality. Committed to sharing his discoveries with others, he has a message of confidence and optimism for his readers. Far from bringing us down, he observes, cancer can transform us; in struggling with it, we will find that because we are more resourceful than we think, we can eventually get the better of fear and defeatism. Having undergone such a transformation himself, he does not now regret having developed cancer; he would absolutely not have wanted to have died the person he was before the cancer recurred. Developing cancer has allowed him to find the true purpose of his life, to know that above all else, everywhere and always, he needs to give all the love that he can. In short, he declares, that is how his death has turned into his life – giving it a power he had never experienced before.

As his death approaches, Gould is undergoing a profound transformation, and is developing a passionate interest in how his life has unfolded. As he reviews the events of his life, he sees a strand of meaning running throughout them. Thinking it over, there is little that he would change; this is his life, and now, it is the time for its meaning to be revealed to him. As he ponders on these last weeks of his life, he notices that he no longer lives in a world of ordinary linear time; since he has no future, it is of no use to him. He realises that in its place, he needs to understand the world in terms that mean something to him as he is now. Finding himself relating to the world around him through his feelings and relationships, he contemplates their movements, their progressions and their changes, taking in the totality of everything, all at once. If he does think of the future, he just hits a rock; on its other side, he is dead. Therefore, he prefers to reach out for the language of spiritual understanding, for the sense of God, for the divine. Living completely in the present as he does, he finds that here and now, there is a place for all things, where all of life's thoughts and feelings seem to circle on themselves.

For Gould, the knowledge that we are going to die can give us a unique sense of meaning in our lives; he believes that this is particularly evident when you know that you are going to die soon. Life is more fulfilling than before, more multi-faceted and ever-changing; he feels as if he can sense the very molecules moving round the room, with more and more of them coming to join the others. Above all, he is aware that death is happening to him at this moment – indeed, at every moment. Metaphysically inspired, he illuminates the way ahead for his family – trying to be strong and to inspire them – though at the same time, he needs their sustaining presence; he declares that he could never get through this experience without their support. Within this extraordinary time, he finds himself in the midst of a paradox; it is he who is dying, but at the same time, it is he who has to show his loved ones the way forward. Intensely aware of everything in and around him, Gould's being in a quasi-mystical state owes little to any organised religion: rather, his sense that he understands, and feels love for all that is around and within him emanates from his own mind. He seems to be endowed with a psychological radiance which relegates his disease to a minor role, and lights up the path ahead for him and for his family. And his intuitive strategy of focusing intensely on the present moment rather than on the point after which he will be dead, might well benefit other people facing death.

Hitchens

For Hitchens, the work of lecturing, debating and writing is everything. Ever since he was laid low by cancer in the midst of a book tour in the summer of 2010, he has delighted in and grasped every possible chance to speak. Unfortunately, this is now beyond his strength; but even as he is living with dying, his greatest solace has been that his friends visit him for just one thing – the opportunity to join him in the joy of conversation. But now, he has a new and alarming problem. Recently, his very ability to talk has come under threat; the other day, without warning, his voice shot up into an infantile, high-pitched peep, and now looks set to vanish completely. And it is not just his voice which is under threat; he explains that with its loss, his whole sense of identity, of who he is, would be endangered. Indeed, thinking about it now, he believes that in his earlier life, he assumed that his voice *was* him, and that he and his voice were one, undivided entity. Having already lost his virility to the treatment, and now, threatened with the castration of this central part of his personality, he feels that he is facing total impotence.

In a final indignity, he is afraid that from once being a master of timing – which is everything in debate – and having lived for the sheer ecstasy of knowing the precise moment to interrupt and top an anecdote, he has been reduced to being listened to 'understandingly'. Accordingly, he can hardly wait to be bombarded with a fusillade of radiation. His objective? – to snatch back the right to freedom of speech. But the disabilities continue to advance; one of the worst is the side effect of peripheral loss of feeling, which threatens him with losing the ability to use his hands to type. Shocked by this development, Hitchens is afraid that if these conditions continue to progress, his will to survive will be relentlessly undermined. After all, writing is not only how he earns a living; it is the very core of his existence.

Hitchens did continue to make notes in his journal; although they became jottings rather than the sentences and paragraphs of his earlier records, he maintained some communication – still characterised by his usual wit and flair – until the day of his death.

Mayne

As he approaches death, Mayne reflects on what has been meaningful in his life:

> [One gift of life is] ... *spiritual*, as we suffer the remorse of reliving and coming to terms with some of our own past actions and motivation; where facing the darkness is an essential part of the healing and ... [we are] restored by ... the 'refining fire'.
>
> (Mayne, p. 36)

For Mayne, our spiritual function includes our psychological processes; its final task in our lives is integration: "Bringing together what is scattered and diverse and forming a satisfying whole; its opposite is segregation, division, alienation .... [I]ntegration brings... peace of mind, whereas the failure to integrate leads to ... depression and even despair" (Mayne, p. 34). In Mayne's view, underneath our everyday concerns and in our deepest selves, our minds are constantly at work, sifting through our life's experience, and assessing and reassessing its meaning:

> The surface mind ... is the 'me' that wants to be in control and fears the unknown .... [and buries] ... all our unresolved baggage .... One [gift] ... of age is that we have the opportunity to lay ... damaging ghosts to rest.
>
> (Mayne, pp. 34–35)

Indeed, he believes that in the interests of resolving conflicts and preparing to die, being controlled by the ego can be beneficially superseded in old age by an increased willingness to ponder the unknown and the disturbing. Quoting again from *Hamlet* but on this occasion, in the hope and expectation that his struggle to understand his experience has not been in vain, he observes: "If, as we grow old and desire with all our being truly to grow as we age, then we may indeed come to understand that 'the readiness is all'" (Mayne, p. 43). In recording this, Mayne is speaking for all of the participants; while the issues they feel the need to understand before they die are personal to them, they do share an intuition that resolving them is the passport to the peace of mind that is an essential aspect of readiness for death.

Taylor

Although she has seemed at times to be caught up, irresolute, and in two minds, Taylor herself feels that her whole life expresses the singular person she feels that she is; indeed, she describes it as the one possible life that she could have lived – as she puts it, as a "singularity saturated with its own oneness" (Taylor, 2016, p. 44). Looking back, she identifies giving birth to her elder son as her first truly important achievement, and once a mother, she knew that she would always put him first; she would watch over and care for him every day until he grew up. Raising her sons has been rewarding beyond words to Taylor, and it makes her happy to see them flourishing even as her own life is on the wane. If this sounds masochistic, in fact it shows that Taylor is constantly surprised and humbled by how much happiness her family has brought her; she finds her own life so much more rewarding than the experience of constant disappointments in each other tolerated by her parents for so many years. In particular, she is grateful to her husband, Shin, for being such a good-natured and caring husband – indeed, she feels that he has helped her to stay sane. In return, believing that she is already indebted to him, she has always tried to avoid letting Shin see that she feels low or troubled. It sounds as if depression has afflicted Taylor for quite some time, and that she has depended on Shin's steadying presence to sustain her through it. Accordingly, she protects Shin from her darker thoughts; for example, as already seen, she is silent at home about having bought a drug with which to euthanise herself if necessary.

In fact, for Taylor, loving someone has never been straightforward. As she recalls those times when she felt most vital and full of life, she realises that for her, fear was often the event that had triggered it, rather than love. In fact, for Taylor, these feelings have always been near neighbours. She had first noticed this as a little girl; with the rest of the family located overseas, she was living alone with her adored mother in Fiji, and would often accompany her to the beach. In the midst of happily watching her mother enjoying the ebb and flow of the water, she would suddenly be seized with terror that her mother might allow a stray breaker to sweep her up, and carry her out to sea. Given her sense early in life that all tender relationships end in tears, Taylor would have been profoundly grateful to Shin for not confirming her long-held assumption that loving someone is bound to be followed by their disappearance. Therein perhaps lies an important reason for her plan to self-euthanise; if that were finally to be enacted, the only disappearance scheduled to take place would be hers.

In fact, reminiscing about her childhood makes Taylor wonder if, however long we live, we ever leave the crucial issues of our early days behind. Initially taking the question literally, she reflects that her cancer is a reminder of a childhood in the sun – an experience she had innocently enjoyed, only to be cruelly reminded of it later. Then, as she recalls T. S. Eliot's lines: '*In the beginning is my end*', she becomes only too aware of its symbolic aspect, that for her, unless she manages to be the first to leave, loving someone has continued to expose her to the fear of losing them. Indeed, when she found her mother in such a parlous state in an institution, her first thought was that she was glad that she already had terminal cancer, and that her future – without her mother – was likely to be limited. In the light of this continuing threat to her emotional equilibrium, perhaps her euthanasia drug also represents an insurance against being confined in an institution like her mother if she should ever become too much for Shin.

In contrast with these catastrophic anxieties, Taylor discovered something as a primary school student which lifted her up then, and carried her forward for the rest of her life; she learnt how to use letters to write words and sentences. From the beginning, it was at the top of her 'must-do' list to acquire the skills of writing. At first, when she noticed how writing traced outlines on paper which only the initiated could understand, it was its enigmatic quality that fascinated her; it was not until later that she became interested in writing as a meaning-maker. For Taylor, as for Diski, this world of symbols and concepts would offer an escape route out of fraught childhood attachments; following the completion of an Arts degree, she became a screenwriter, with a life of her own.

Meaningfulness in life and in dying: Summary

There are two main themes in the participants' contributions to this category. Firstly, every participant writes about the central importance to them of loving and being loved, and apart from Diski's rancour towards the oncologist and Hitchens' towards Christians, very little about animosity. Although Diski never mentions the word 'love' except to query its having any relevance to her, she actually writes lovingly about her grandchildren; Gould makes a commitment to giving love – especially to his family, but seemingly to all creation – as his ultimate purpose in life; Hitchens' writing and lecturing are so adored that he believes without it, the will to live might well desert him; Mayne is dedicated to spiritual contemplation, greatly loves his family and friends, and believes that God loves him unconditionally; finally, Taylor dearly loves her husband and sons, and has always adored her mother.

Secondly, every participant writes about the importance to them of their creativity which, in the sense of imparting something of themselves to succeeding generations, is linked for four participants – Gould, Hitchens, Mayne and Taylor – with experiencing a touch of immortality. Gould believes his destiny to be eternal transfiguration; his earthly responsibility is to educate present and future cancer sufferers to face down their fear of death and become stronger for it. As a believer, Mayne imagines eternity with God, and he wants his memoir to offer comfort and empathy for future lonely sufferers when the going is hard. Hitchens wants to stockpile iconoclastic weapons to protect the vulnerable into the future against the dangerous nonsense peddled by the begodded. On publishing her first novel, Taylor dreams of a moment of immortality if someone reading her books pauses to think of her as their author. However, although Diski's meticulous research and her massive creative output were central to her life prior to the cancer diagnosis, her writing has been experienced as a way of expressing and maintaining herself; accordingly, for Diski, it dies with her. For these dying people, it is love, and for four of them, a creativity which they hope will nourish others in the future, that have been the most meaningful things in their lives; the same treasured qualities continue to sustain them through the travails of dying.

In Chapter 2, *Death as enigma*. Part III: *Sequestration of the dying*, organisational analyst, Hugh Willmott, argues that when death approaches, we find ourselves exposed to an awareness of the insignificant nature of the projects which we have depended upon for our sense of immortal self-identity. Therefore, when death is in the offing, we are left with an overwhelming sense of confusion and insignificance, because of "the projected loss of ... our socially-constructed sense of self-identity, that arises simultaneously with participation in modern institutions" (Willmott, 2000, p. 658). However, the findings discussed above do not support this view. The four participants who became capable of accepting death with composure reported that their sense of self-identity remained strong to the end; only one, Diski, who unlike the others, had suffered years of severe psychiatric illness when young, experienced dying as destructive to her sense of self-identity, personally and as a writer. Certainly, the other four participants did derive part of their sense of self-identity from membership of their calling, and they did hope to have made a contribution to the welfare of others which would continue after they had died. But it was a modest hope, not one which sought a grandiose immortality through identification with their professional institutions; as participant Michael Mayne put it, their writings were offered as a last gift to the world: "'speaking what we feel, not what we ought to say'.... [A] small – and sometimes quite risky – act of love" (Mayne, 2006, p. 246).

The participants were in substantial agreement about what had been most meaningful to them in life and in dying. Firstly, every participant wrote about the crucial importance of love. Secondly, every participant wrote about the peerless value to them of their creativity and – apart from Diski – its role in their sense of making a contribution to future generations.

At this point, the participants are exploring their understanding of and attitudes to death, and what they imagine dying will be like; all but one of them are preparing to meet it with acceptance. The fifth participant, Diski, is fearful that she cannot 'do' dying, or ever find it in herself to accept her death.

The last of three chapters of the participants' narrative, Chapter 7, *Acceptance*, examines the psychological work involved as the participants grapple with readying themselves for finally letting go.

References

Diski, J. (2016). *In gratitude*. London and New York: Bloomsbury Publishing.

Fielding, Henry. (1751/2017). *Amelia, volume I* (Paperback). Scotts Valley, CA: CreateSpace Independent Publishing Platform.

Gould, P. (2013). *When I die: Lessons from the death zone*. London: Abacus, Little, Brown Book Group.

Hitchens, C. E. (2012). *Mortality*. New York, Boston, MA: Twelve Books.

Mayne, M. C. O. (2006). *The enduring melody*. London: Darton, Longman & Todd.

Taylor, C. (2016). *Dying: A memoir*. Melbourne: Text Publishing.

Willmott, H. (2000). Death. So what? Sociology, sequestration and emancipation. *The Sociological Review, 48*(4), 649–665. Retrieved from https://onlinelibrary.wiley.com/doi/abs/10.1111/1467-954X.00237

7 Acceptance

Introduction

Now entering the final phase of their illness and with death coming ever closer, the participants realise intuitively that preparing for death will require them to identify and sort out the most fundamental of their outstanding conflicts – whether internal to them, or between them and other people. For them all, the relevant issues are longstanding, and have resisted attempts to resolve them for many years. Further, in a type of death-bed confession, three of them reveal that their consciences are burdened with actions they have taken, or negative attitudes they have hidden, for which they need to find a way to forgive themselves before they die. Part I of the following chapter examines these and other aspects of their struggle to be ready for, and to accept death as the natural end to life, while Part II discusses the final thoughts recorded in each participant's memoir.

Part I is further divided into a number of sub-sections:

Part I. Working towards acceptance (*Resolution of conflicts; Confessions; How dying is prepared for)*
Part II. Final thoughts

Part I. Working towards acceptance (*Resolution of conflicts; Confessions; How dying is prepared for*)

Resolution of conflicts

All participants contribute to this sub-category; Diski, Mayne and Taylor are concerned with internal conflicts, while the issues to be resolved by Hitchens and Gould are between them and significant others.

Diski: 'I can't do dying' – The fear of imploding

From the age of fifteen to nineteen and at her invitation, Diski lived in the home of the writer, Doris Lessing; her inability to escape from the dominant

DOI: 10.4324/9781003392088-7

Lessing's belittling attitude to her preoccupied Diski throughout her life. She had been at boarding school with Lessing's son Peter, and although he was only a little older than Diski, Peter had told his mother that Diski had nobody to care for her and that she needed help; he had instructed his mother to take Diski in. A moody and out-of-control adolescent, once installed, Diski found that her status in the Lessing household and how long she was to be there could not be clarified, and she was never sure of being welcome. As she acknowledges: "I've always been prepared to use extreme measures ... to put an end to uncertainty in my life" (Diski, 2016, p.118). Accordingly, having agonised over the question of her standing with Lessing for months, Diski finally asked her about it: "'You hadn't met me when you wrote to me ... [and] I'm really grateful. But now I'm here and you've known me ... If you don't really like me, there's nowhere you could send me back to is there?'" (Diski, p. 76). Lessing did not reply, and Diski became anxious:

> The silence remained ... long enough to ... frighten me ... Doris ... walked out of the room ... the front door banged shut as she left the house ... I had no idea what had happened ... I was terrified.
>
> (Diski, p. 77)

The next morning, Diski found a letter to her from Lessing on the kitchen table: "What I had done last night was unforgivable. She couldn't remember ... anyone trying to blackmail her emotionally as I had done" (Diski, p. 78). Diski was now sure that Lessing did not like her, and that to win her over, she must appear more willing to comply with Lessing's directives on how she should behave: "We continued with ... the upgrading of my overemotional tendencies, proving myself a good bet in the making something of myself" (Diski, p. 82).

Since Diski had been sexually abused by her parents as a small child, her relationship with the Lessings reactivated an earlier trauma; the assumption created then – that she was entitled to exist only as the plaything of a powerful couple – had never been overturned. From her adolescence on, believing that her parents disliked her, Diski saw little of them; in any case, by then, her father was living elsewhere with his second wife. Then, having been cast aside by her parents, she was suddenly offered a home; as if magically parachuted into her life, the Lessings may have initially seemed to her to be the paragon of a parental couple, everything that her actual parents were not. Little wonder, then, that she endowed the sophisticated and intellectual Doris Lessing with the power finally to make everything right by accepting her, or to bring her down by being disappointed in her. And now, having at last exposed her anxiety about being unwanted to Lessing, she had been comprehensively rejected; in the equivalent of crawling away, she took it that she would have to try to intuit Lessing's expectations of her, and comply with them, if she wanted to remain in Lessing's home. At barely sixteen, with nowhere else to go, Diski's options were limited, leaving her little alternative but to submit to the terms Lessing laid down. Unfortunately, Lessing never recognised in her question about where she stood, that Diski was asking her to consider whether or not she might have an authentic self which would be worth fostering. To take a snapshot of their relationship: When Diski was sent by Lessing to a highly-regarded London clinic for psychotherapy, the psychiatrist asked to meet Lessing to talk about Diski's difficulties. According to Diski, after the interview, Lessing returned home fuming: "He told her that my depression was due to my not being in a real relationship with her ... I couldn't behave the way most adolescents behaved with their real family, knowing there would always be a reprieve". Clearly nettled, Lessing demanded that Diski concur: "'You don't feel you can't say anything because you're not my real daughter, do you?' ... I ... said 'No', as insincerely as I could manage. 'Of course not,' Doris said, 'the man's an idiot'" (Diski, pp. 220–221). Diski's attendance at the clinic was discontinued.

A further vexed issue concerned Diski's wish to become a writer. Although she was living in a household frequented by the *literati*, Diski's potential as a writer was not recognised by Lessing, and was actively resented by Peter: "Years later, a friend told me that ... Peter had said to him that: 'The worst thing that could happen to me would be if Jenny became a successful novelist'" (Diski, p. 202). In fact, Lessing wanted Diski to go to University; as Diski saw it: "I had been saved to amount to something. I wasn't sure I was up to it, but I tried to play along" (Diski, p. 80). Mired in a triangular relationship with the Lessings for the next fifty years, Diski devotes almost half of her memoir to its scrutiny, concluding: "I believe Doris took a grave risk with three people's lives, and I can't really untangle the strands that might tell me why" (Diski, p. 204).

It must surely be very difficult to accept dying – ceasing to exist – from a position of having never been endowed with the right to exist as oneself in the first place. Such a right has to be bestowed on one by someone who has the power to confer it – usually parents or their substitutes – or at least, not denied by the enforcement on the child of their own expectations. Given her experience of being used as a sexualised plaything by her parents and finally abandoned, Diski urgently needed to join a family group which would prioritise her need to be recognised and valued for herself. From the outset, however, the Lessings did not seem to conceptualise their project of rescuing her in that way. Indeed, although she had read some texts on mental disturbance and according to Diski, thought that she was quite informed on the subject, Lessing could have had no idea either of the depth and complexity of Diski's psychological problems, or of how dire her circumstances were at the time of Lessing's intervention. She did know that Diski was in hospital following a suicide attempt by overdose, but she did not seem to know, or to have understood in any depth, its immediate cause or longer-term background.

Before being taken on by Lessing, Diski had been expelled from her sponsored place at a Council boarding school for escaping at night to meet boys; with nowhere else to go, the runaway Diski had sought refuge with her mother in her one-bedroom Council flat in Hove. They had to share the one available bed, and during the night, Diski's mother tried to fondle her vulva; on being shrieked at, she protested: "But you're still my little girl!". Diski went to another room, and in quiet despair, took an overdose of her mother's Nembutal. It was during her ensuing stay in hospital after having had her stomach pumped, that Diski received a letter from Lessing containing an offer of a home, and the financial support to allow her to return to school. Following an appreciative letter of provisional acceptance of her offer from Diski and only one meeting with her and her mother, armed with the go-ahead from the doctor who was responsible for Diski during her stay in hospital, Lessing took Diski into her home.

To the adults involved, this had seemed to offer the adolescent Diski the opportunity of a lifetime. For Diski, however, there was a catch; she had no idea why she had been taken up by the Lessings, and had not been invited to trial how all parties would experience her living with them. In effect, she was being strongly encouraged – even pressed – to commit herself to a leap in the dark. As a consequence, she never saw herself as having entered as a chosen and welcome member of the Lessing household; rather than being liked and wanted for herself, she felt like a charity case, a 'foister-child'. Demonstrating how vulnerable she was to being put in a role similar to the one originally imposed on her by her parents, Diski had understood that she should go along with the project and try to please, while at the same time, remaining convinced that there was nothing else that she could possibly do that would justify her presence there.

Typically, although someone in that position may complain about particular incidents in their day-to-day lives, they do not usually question their acceptance of the role *per se* and its part in the family system as a whole; that such a meta-reality even exists is ordinarily beyond their awareness. Moreover, showing disidentification or unhappiness with their prescribed role carries the likelihood of fatally displeasing the taskmaster. Inchoate fears of doing this might include being cast out forever, or being overtaken by feelings of disintegration, of falling to pieces. In order to survive and in a limited way, to prosper, Diski was setting herself up in a kind of alternate reality, in which she had no origins; this allowed her to construe herself as a one-off self-invention, like a character from one of her brilliant and eccentric novels. However, when thrust into a socially endorsed role – for example, "Lessing's sponsored charge", or later, "terminally ill patient" – she suffered from overwhelming embarrassment or shame. Perhaps this was symptomatic of a sense of radical dissonance that she experienced on making an enforced re-entry into the seceded-from ordinary world where, having had only provisional membership, she would have to face the rejection, perhaps ridicule, of its authorised inhabitants.

Returning to Diski's present life circumstance as a terminally-ill patient: Being constantly engaged in the writing life as she has been for thirty years is no longer an option for the dying Diski; lacking a sense of future and the energy to fuel it, she has lost the motivation to write anything other than her memoir. Moreover, unable to resolve her conflicts, she can find no rest from the fear of dying in torment. However, because she feels a unique tenderness towards her grandchildren, she does experience some respite – a kind of painful joy – whenever they come to visit. Now, though she does not seem to recognise it in the midst of the pain that she is suffering about their loss, this unique outpouring of tenderness for her grandchildren may have the potential to be redemptive.

The Oxford Dictionaries' definition of 'redemption' applies in secular as well as religious contexts: "The action of saving or being saved from sin, error or evil". (Retrieved 20/11/18, from https://en.oxforddictionaries.com/definition/redemption)

Since the definition uses both active and passive voices, it is implied that although an individual may consciously seek redemption, it may equally be conferred upon them by circumstance, or as a result of something else that they have experienced or done. Accordingly, the suggestion that Diski's spontaneous tenderness towards her grandchildren might potentially be redemptive does not require her to be aware of it. Arguably, however, finding redemption does seem to imply that the protagonist realises that they have fallen from grace; that Diski knows how full of black thoughts she is will be clear from her observations in *Confessions,* below; for example:

> I'm not genuinely grateful at all. Not in that dark place where I am a naughty, angry child. I can't feel genuinely anything much because that train left the platform before I knew it was there ... [Some] can see only the bleak side of anything good or innocuous ... a world of my own making.
>
> (Diski, pp. 205–206)

If this is right, for Diski to benefit from it does not require her to identify what the redemptive experience should be; what matters is whether the experience has changed her in a humanising way. Perhaps it has; from having avowedly been incapable of it until now, she has conceived a spontaneous and unconditional love for her grandchildren. She notes, but never regrets, the price she has to pay in their prospective loss.

Diski: 'Doing dying' – The fear of imploding: Summary

Recalling the discussion of Diski's fears about dying in Chapter 6, Sub-set: *Imagining dying: 'Doing dying':* "In Diski's nightmare scenario, we may not know how to 'do' dying, but we will have to go ahead anyway, and be mangled by it". It is not clear just what Diski fears will overtake her, and it is possible that she could not explain it any further herself. Arguably, however, though perhaps similarly unaware of it, Diski, and other individuals who share her dilemma, are unconsciously terrified not so much of ceasing to exist while dying but rather, of ceasing to exist as coherent beings while they are still alive; the two imagined catastrophes have become conflated.

In this connection, a comparison can be made between Diski's fears of a meltdown of consciousness being brought on by dying, and remarks on the same subject by Taylor and by me. Explaining why she wanted to write a memoir about dying, Taylor wrote that she wanted to create an outline of her death, so that both she and others could see clearly what the experience was like for her, and secondly, to make dying bearable for herself (see Chapter 5, p. 4). My contribution is the observation in which I 'heard' that: "Everything will be fine" (see Chapter 1, p. 4). Arguably, the underlying issue involved here is whether or not an individual believes that inhabiting a dying body will destroy the integrity of their mind and spirit. After a struggle, Taylor and I both understood that although we had been diagnosed as dying from a ravaging disease, our minds would remain sane and in charge of the enterprise. However, alone among the participants – though Mayne and Hitchens at times feared it – Diski persistently believed that her mind's control of her organism as a whole was slipping away, and with it, her holding herself together as a coherent being. As if trapped in a snare, Diski was caught in a quandary; although her mind was increasingly filled with tormenting thoughts, for her, the loss of its hegemony could only spell catastrophe. And the more she struggled against her fate, the tighter the grip of the snare became.

Gould: Reckonings

While Gould and his wife, Gail, have a strong and loving relationship, it is not free from unresolved differences, and as the time that Gould has left has now become radically foreshortened, Gail seems to have realised that she must raise an important issue with him before it is too late. As Gould later recalls this encounter, Gail confronted him with how he had demolished her home-making over the years; pleasing himself at her expense, and regardless of how many of her lovingly created and beautiful family homes he destroyed in the process, he had persisted in moving the family on from one home to another to suit himself and his work. Suddenly realising the enormity of his self-absorption, Gould believes that it was only because of the imminence of his death that he could stop and listen, and give Gail's charge the attention it deserved. Without delay, he let her know that he could see how wrong his behaviour had been, and how remorseful he felt, and was forgiven. From that time on, he believes, their relationship moved to a new level, where it has remained.

Apparently, Gould had never before paid attention to Gail's exasperation, but evidently, while she had capitulated until now and life had gone on as usual, there had been a gathering resentment on her part. Her challenging Gould at this point is risky; if unresolved, it could leave them both distressed and alone when they most need to be united. As it turned out, however, their relationship was repaired and enriched by the interchange.

It may not be unusual for the dying and those close to them to review the events of a lifetime and to seek to resolve conflicts, but Gould is the only participant to report a significant clash with a loved one; his account demonstrates how constructive a final reckoning can be. Indeed, Gould believes that only his terminal illness could provide the impetus for such a major reckoning. As well as its having created the pause in daily life to allow Gail's challenge to him to be aired, his imminent death has finally disposed him to pay attention to it.

Gould: Reckonings: Summary

Gould believes that death gives life meaning; this is a much-debated philosophical point, but it is made by no other participant. Now, while raising grievances in order to effect reconciliation with others before dying is advocated by some, Gould is the only participant to report having experienced it. As it happens, Gould's narrative shows that he and Gail were both strong individuals who valued their relationship profoundly; if these criteria were not met, a confrontation might be risky, and the outcome a less happy one.

Mayne: A father for all seasons

To Mayne, dynamic psychology is an integral part of spiritual understanding: "At the level of my unconscious all my experiences exist timelessly ... [M]y unique story [is told] ... by linking together memory and imagination ... I can gather lost moments and experiences, and ... hold them as one" (Mayne, 2006, p. 31). He has a rare insight into himself, and from the initial cancer diagnosis on, he works steadily on resolving his conflicts about his relationship to father-figures, including God. Unable to steady himself through prayer when initially diagnosed, Mayne remains concerned about how to sustain contact with God:

> I see prayer as ... the conscious uniting with that deep centre of life and healing of me and those ... I love and who love me ... [and those] who will treat me ... [Tapping] ... into the creative source of life itself.
>
> (Mayne, p. 55)

However, he must add: "I felt held, right up to the morning of the operation ... but in the dark days that followed I felt nothing at times but the darkness (as Jesus ... felt ... in the Garden of Gethsemane)" (Mayne, p. 80). But he believes that: "The 'feelings' were caused by the poison in my veins. The reality is ... that I was ... vigorously upheld in God's presence" (Mayne, p. 81). However generated, the ability to make a strong recovery from dark feelings is one of Mayne's most valuable assets; it allows him to move through confronting issues to an enduring conclusion: "I have learned that, while God may often seem remote ... in a crisis God's grace works through the kindness and thoughtfulness of the countless people whose lives we have touched" (Mayne, p. 245).

As the treatment becomes more painful, disfiguring and destructive to his quality of life, he finds that his previously favoured image of an always tenderly smiling Jesus has to change, in order to accommodate this new reality; he becomes aware that this need for a change of heart is connected with his fatherless childhood. At first, he had resisted it:

> When I retired ... one of my gifts was an icon ... [I]t was a stern, unsmiling Christ ... [and] ... at times like the present I yearn for a more tender gaze. (Perhaps that's my strange fatherless, rather lonely childhood speaking).
>
> (Mayne, p. 97)

But then, he understands something for the first time: "My icon suggests the Gethsemane Christ ... who shares the suffering. That's the Christ I need now" (Mayne, pp. 97–98). He understands that, although Jesus had experienced pain and evil, and when on the cross, had even felt abandoned by God, he had always regained his belief in, and capacity for fatherly love. Grasping the core of this mystery gives Mayne strength: "Ultimately [Jesus] ... did not question the good purpose of God. He felt the full force of these questions, but they were contained within his overriding concept of the fatherly love of the Father" (Mayne, p. 100). As he thinks about this more multi-faceted Jesus, his mind moves to his suicided father; though he strives to be compassionate, Mayne has not been able to understand and accept his father's actions: "My own father's suicide ...was ... for my mother and me, an act of betrayal ... of trust. And my mother ... often made emotional demands on me which could paralyse my own emotions and inhibit my response" (Mayne, pp. 118–119). As Jesus was deserted by his father, so too was Mayne; effectively parentless at only three years old, he was left to cope with his tragically widowed and at times, suffocatingly needy mother. Having by now become aware that, like most of us, he will always have to take account of a well of negative and painful feelings within him, Mayne discards the tenderly-smiling Jesus as unidimensional, and turns instead to the Gethsemane Jesus as his father-figure.

Mayne's capacity for such a profound change of attitude is cause for some wonderment. He appears to have had an unusual ability to contact and interact with his unconscious mind, and because he had the moral courage and emotional intelligence to do it, he was able to receive and understand its wordless communications. A significant example of this occurred while he was mulling over the relationship with his father. The episode concerned – described in detail in the next paragraph – happened at Easter, a time in which Jesus' suffering on the cross, and his fears of having been forsaken by God, would have been a potent symbol of Mayne's struggles with what he had experienced as his father's abandoning him. During this time, he had a remarkable encounter with himself, in which a cluster of unconscious processes broke through his defences and confronted him in all their vividness and power. He emphasises that he was wide awake throughout the experience, that it was not a dream but rather, a waking hallucination, a display of intimidating imagery over which he had no control. Of course, that such a decompensation occurred in his normal waking state would almost certainly have been partly due to the potent drugs that he had been given, but their meaningful import for him, and the fact that, although he trembled, he did not try to look away, are a tribute to Mayne's continuing fortitude in his search for his own existential truth. In what follows, he describes what took place.

One night, as he got into bed, he found that he had lost control of his mind, that he had gone "completely dotty":

> I began talking not just jumbled-up words, but nonsense words, gobbledegook. I knew I was doing so but could do nothing to stop it [and] ... my doctor was off-duty. The second stage was to start visualising individuals with acute vividness – every mole and wrinkle. None of them spoke: they simply arrived at the end of our bed, their eyes growing larger and more accusing. Over the next five days (all through Easter) the numbers grew, night and day; sometimes the small bedroom was crammed with up to twenty of them, all staring me down, and I felt too ill to get up ... The ... room was decorated in a variety of exotic fashions ... and I would be looking down at it from different angles of the ceiling. There was, I discovered, one simple way of banishing these visitors: by holding their gaze and blinking hard. But it only worked for the current ones, and immediately others would appear. I grew fairly weak, and at times – such as when I found myself kneeling on the end of the bed ... and staring myself down – quite frightened too ... There was nothing dream-like about the experience: I was wide awake throughout ... There were voices, and music ... The duty doctor came and took me off all medication ... it was a relief to see ... our GP, back on Tuesday, who re-prescribed.
>
> (p. 234)

While suspending incredulity over items in this account which may seem hard to take on board – perhaps, that the episode lasted for five days – nonetheless, many elements of it seem relevant to Mayne's struggle to find peace over the emotional legacy left to him by his parents. At the outset of the episode, he seems to be set up for punishment; he is brought down by no longer being able to make sense of his own thoughts and then, trapped, as an endless stream of accusing images, spilling out of his unconscious mind, begins crowding in on him. Most threatening of all is an image which is a facsimile of himself – perhaps the incarnation of a reproachful, finger-pointing conscience, or an imaginary, unloved father. Evidently finding him guilty of some dire sin for which, in their eyes, he has not atoned, his unknown accusers seem intent upon overwhelming him with their sheer numbers; evidently, he has been convicted, and seems to be about to be punished. And yet, throughout his life, and despite his disillusionment with them, he has tried to maintain the memory of his tragically disappointing parents as kindly as he can, and by becoming a priest, he has accepted that he has a contingent obligation to care for, and to try to redeem, anyone else who might need it. Moreover, he has acquiesced in a further requirement of him, that he should always pardon the deficient, including those who have personally let him down; earlier in this narrative, occasions were recorded when he had been painfully failed by his doctors, but he had reflected nothing but approval back to them. Indeed, he seemed to feel obliged to be *their* always smiling icon. Evidently, however, at the time of these accusatory hallucinations, none of this has redeemed him.

Perhaps in his depths, he has a well of anger about having never felt free to repudiate the role of unworthy penitent imposed on him by his own inner critic, merged with the father-figure within; if so, righteous anger comes to his rescue and powers his response now. Standing by the integrity of his own emotions at last, and despite the continuing barrage of reproaches, he stares back at his accusers, blinks them into vaporising and by a sheer assertion of will, forces them to disappear; in so doing, he lets them know that what he feels is not trivial and expendable, and that it is not only their feelings that count, or are real. He does not offer, or demand apologies or forgiveness, nor does he counter-attack. From what he has revealed of himself so far, it is probable that what he would like to see is mutual forbearance, an acknowledgement of failures and transgressions all round, together with an attempt first to understand, rather than immediately to invalidate or condemn.

Soon after this breakthrough, Mayne received his terminal diagnosis; he notes that receiving the news did not alter anything that he had written so far. Accordingly, it is timely to remind ourselves of the tremulous Mayne of the initial diagnosis phase, troubled by his inability to feel in touch with God. Now, however, it is a resolute and steady Mayne who observes: "I find myself saying more and more: 'I can do all things through Christ who strengthens me'" (Mayne, p. 249), even though: "There is … shock in hearing it spelled out so finally, and part of me wants to weep and feels nothing but fear and dismay" (Mayne, p. 250). However, he and his wife have come to the decision to reject further chemotherapy: "I don't intend to spin things out … [T]hese last days [are about] … not the *amount* of time left to me but its *quality*" (Mayne, p. 246). He is coming to the end of his pilgrimage; he has become his own man: "Graham, our GP … visits … I say how grateful we are that we are being cared for by such a good team. 'And don't forget', he replies, 'that you're the team leader'" (Mayne, p. 249).

Even when just recently diagnosed with cancer, Mayne had experienced intuitions of mortality; at the same time, he had felt that God's presence was remote. During the long nights of pain and drug-induced hallucinations that he endured in his first surgery, his experience of losing his sense of connection with God when he most needed it had left him afraid that at any time, it could be broken. Now, it might be thought that finding his faith so difficult to access as he faced death was so intolerable to Mayne that he had been obliged to switch off his doubts about God's love, but this does not appear to be the case. Rather, he seems to have allowed himself to be carried along on a profound psychic mission of which – though he experienced a number of insights on the way – he never consciously identified the nature or the objective. However, as a consequence of it he made peace with the memory of his father, recognised himself as belonging to the Gethsemane Jesus' congregation and finally, became a wise father to himself, and to his family.

Mayne: A father for all seasons: Summary

A forward-moving narrative seems to have developed in Mayne's unconscious mind with which he seemed intuitively to know how to interact. At times – as when his choice of icon was challenged – this narrative emerged in his consciousness, and required him to analyse and radically change the attitudes of a lifetime. Experiences of feeling carried towards one's destiny when dying are not uncommon; Mayne would probably have attributed his own to God's plan for him.

Taylor: To be or not to be

As recorded in the previous chapter, in *Imagining dying*, Taylor is troubled by guilt at failing her adored mother at the end of her life. Now facing her own death, she takes her mother's advice and joins Exit International, but she goes further; for use if dying leads to her autonomy being threatened, she has also acquired a euthanasia drug online. From then on, it seems, she often struggles with the pros and cons of taking this drug, generally declaring that, even if she never uses it, she retains it because it gives her control over her destiny. In particular, as long as she has the drug secreted, together with her suicide note, she can rest assured that she can always find some remedy for the fear of becoming totally dependent that hangs over her.

Yet, given that, in her account below, in *How dying is prepared for: How it ends for each participant*, para. 4, she has for some time been as helpless as an infant, it is puzzling that in explanation of obtaining the drug, she continues to refer to it as a means of taking control by suicide in the event of becoming dependent and helpless. Further, in the previous chapter, *Imagining dying*, and apparently in contradiction of her oft-repeated assertion that possessing the drug protects her from a horrible death, Taylor has declared that perhaps the real reason for her reluctance to take her own life is that suicide is so dangerous. Indeed, words fail her in the face of the terrifying abyss that is death. Though clearly unwilling to kill herself, she seems to lack the ability to abandon the drug, and call off the suicide plan. Perhaps she does not know, or cannot articulate, what her real reason for retaining the drug is.

Perhaps recapitulating her story will help to make some sense of this confusing picture. When as a child Taylor had lived for some years in Fiji, her airline pilot father was often absent and her older siblings were at boarding school in Australia; as a consequence, she and her mother were left for long periods on their own. It was a blissful time for Taylor, lazing in the sun in often wordless companionship with her mother, but with no one to come between them and provide the impetus needed for Taylor to develop a separate sense of self, communication skills, and an independent life and friends. It is possible that, in a regressed state brought on by facing death at the end of years of terminal illness, Taylor had drifted back into a comforting identification with that blissful, at-one, mother-daughter symbiosis. If this is right, feeling as if she were part of her mother, and her mother part of her, might also have carried a threat; she could not always separate her own experience from her mother's, and therefore, her own dying from how her mother had died, abandoned and alone. Indeed, being so identified with her mother, as noted earlier, Taylor regularly finds herself in two minds.

In one, she is her autonomous adult self, and although weak and dependent, she is cared for at home by her husband and visiting medical professionals; there is no need for her to self-euthanise. In the other, however, she is at one with her mother, made vulnerable by having a potentially unmanageable illness, to being abandoned to the neglect and helplessness of life in an institution. Moreover, again like her mother, she has no support from her adult children to help her to die. If she does decide to die by euthanasia, she will have to be prepared to do the job herself, and to do it alone.

Yet, since she had dementia and no longer spoke, her mother could never have asked Taylor to help her to die; hence, Taylor's sin could not have been a failure to help her mother to die when asked to do so. Rather, her sin was surely that, in her mother's hour of greatest need, she had deserted her. As a consequence, the manner of her mother's death offered the dying Taylor neither a model, nor the image of a loyally cared-for loved one with whom to identify. In fact, her mother's death appears to have haunted her as the worst kind of death imaginable. It is likely that, in the grip of an ensuant unconscious fear of being punished for neglecting her mother by first, losing her protection, and then, undergoing the same kind of death herself, Taylor equipped herself with the means to euthanise herself. However, as the likelihood of being abandoned to die in an institution like her mother gradually receded, she found herself released from this particular trap, only to then find herself lost in a psychological vacuum. In her final weeks, with no positive model to embrace in how her mother had died, she was left alone, and obliged to find an alternative path to death. But with no longer any purpose to serve, the drug's one-time importance to Taylor simply faded away.

Of course, Taylor's symbiotic relationship with her mother goes well beyond the province of her dying. Indeed, at this stage in Taylor's life, it still involves most of her inner world. By way of illustration, it is possible that the frequent abrupt changes of tone in Taylor's narrative that were noted earlier reflect the drift between her identification with a more autonomous adult self who speaks in a mature way, and an at-oneness with her child-mother co-mingled self, who often speaks quite brusquely. At such times, Taylor sounds like an irritably anxious child adopting an offhand manner but in fact, trying to capture the elusive attention of a mother who might at any time be carried off, not so much by a stray wave, as by something unpredictable that Taylor has intuited in her nature. This kind of double-agency message is seen in Taylor's direction to her husband that he can "toss me (her ashes) out when he is ready", rather than speaking as a mature woman might, when trying to put sensitive words to an unthinkable reality – the prospect of her husband becoming the custodian of her cremated body, and obliged to see to its disposal. Shortly thereafter, she seems to 'come to', and starts to think about how she might be able to help her husband and sons to plan for this potentially difficult day.

In order to resolve this fusion and confusion before she dies, Taylor would need to separate her present self out from the identities within, acknowledge that her mother has been dead these ten years, and let her go. To achieve so much change in such a short time could well be out of the question. Fortunately, however, Taylor has a well-developed creative imagination to draw on, which might allow her to create an alternative path to a peaceful death.

Taylor: To be or not to be: Summary

At this point, Taylor remains suspended between her adult self and a child/mother self from whom she needs to find release. As she has so far been unable either to resolve conflicts or to identify an emergent third position on which to base her decisions – including the manner of her departure from this life – it remains to be seen how she will move out of her dilemma, and ready herself for death. In the meantime, however, she refers to the euthanasia drug less and less often; perhaps this is a first sign that she is experiencing a dawning intuition of a quite different path to her death.

Hitchens: I do not recant

Not a fan of self-analysis, the antitheistic Hitchens' conflict was with those Christian believers who were jubilant that he had cancer, which they thought served him right; some even began to spread a rumour that a terrified Hitchens had recanted his antitheism on his deathbed. Wanting to create a permanent rebuttal of these insinuations, Hitchens devoted the first chapter of his memoir to restating his warnings about the dangers of becoming captive to the misleading nonsense of religious believers (Hitchens, 2012).

Resolution of conflicts: Summary

For the dying, the foreseeable future is about to end in the ultimate bereavement – the loss of everything they care about. According to a group of academic social workers specialising in loss and bereavement, theory and empirical evidence both suggest that people suffering loss who have unresolved regrets experience lower levels of well-being than do those who resolve them (Torges, Stewart and Nolen-Hoeksma, 2008, p. 169). Certainly, all of the present participants do experience an intuitively compelling need to resolve lingering conflicts before they die. Only one participant, Diski, has so far been unable to resolve her dilemma, and for Taylor, it is still hanging in the balance; but the other three have been successful in doing so.

Resolution of intrapsychic conflicts does not seem to require a clear identification of what is at issue in the same way that the external confrontations facing Gould and Hitchens did. Rather, the possibility of their resolution seems to depend on how the individual interacts with the signs of the conflict when they surface, as in Mayne's dilemma over his choice of icon, Diski's over appealing to her oncologist to help her to connect with her terminal condition, and Taylor's over using the euthanising drug. It is not possible to draw general conclusions about the percentage of the dying who might be capable of resolving final conflicts from a sample of this size, whose members might, moreover, be atypical in their ability to articulate and work through conflictual issues. It is suggested, however, that dying individuals may often be faced with significant conflicts to resolve before they die, and that, as a lack of resolution may impede their acceptance of dying, they may need informal or perhaps, professional assistance.

Confessions

Deathbed confessions are popular in fiction, but they are recorded by only three participants – Diski, Gould and Taylor.

Diski: Ingratitude

Near the end of her memoir, Diski addresses the title of her book, *In gratitude*:

> In all honesty ... I'm not genuinely grateful at all. Not in that dark place where I am a naughty, angry child. I can't feel genuinely anything much because that train left the platform before I knew it was there, or I slept, as it stopped and started off again without a thought for its sleepy passenger ... Perhaps I *was* asleep when the shards of glass dropped from the playful cherubims' hands and fell arbitrarily into the

> eyes or hearts of some, but only some. Broken mirrors falling through the sky, to change the hearts and minds of a few people so that they can see only the bleak side of anything good or innocuous ... That must be my sliver of looking glass, reflecting a place where everything is not what it seems, a world of my own making, of tickling death and then hiding between my own legs, as one hid behind one's mother's in shame or anxiety. Goblin. Hobgoblin. There once was an ugly duckling. *There* was a promise for those who saw the world as it really was. But promises aren't always kept and I can't tolerate unfulfilled promises. My head is full of dark, terrorising tales... Collected or made up on the spot. ... The stories never run out, especially the 'real' ones, the ones that actually happened ... When [elephant's teeth] ... run out – the ones planted before birth in the world – the elephant starves to death. The wicked cruelty of nature. Always another trick up its sleeve. Some of us will suffocate, some will starve. Some will spend their days waiting for the end of the story. I guess some people don't. Certainly, I doubt that elephants fret about the way the end will come.
>
> (Diski, pp. 205–206)

Diski acknowledges feeling the angry defiance of a child who is disappointed in and contemptuous of a hypocritical adult world. Her talk of gratitude to Doris Lessing – as expressed in the last section, *Resolution of conflicts* – now sounds more like a 'charity case' pretending to be compliant, while secretly feeling only fear and resentment. However, although she herself expresses no sadness, there is truth and pathos in her observation that the capacity-to-genuinely-feel train had left the platform before she knew it was there. She goes on to describe her revenge on her betrayers – a 'bleaking-out' of everything apparently good or innocuous, and a refusal to accept the deceptive appearance of an agreeable society. In referring to "tickling death and then hiding between my own legs, as one hid behind one's mother's in shame or anxiety", she seems to be drawing on an intuition that the sexual abuse she endured as a child lies behind her killing off everything that proclaims itself as good. But trapped as she is in a system of abuser and abused, there is the danger of killing off what actually *is* good, of doing to others what was done to her. For example, it would have been central to her disappointment in Doris Lessing that while she had taken Lessing's invitation to be a commitment to care for her, it seemed to her that Lessing did not even want to get to know her. Arguably, however, Diski is here being hypocritical herself. If, as the abandoned child, she had become the object of special attention, she might well have considered Lessing obsequious; her response would probably have been scathing. Having avoided this fate, the supremely confident Lessing unfortunately could not offer her anything more sustaining – throughout her dealings with Diski, she seemed to show little empathy or sensitivity – and Diski was left dangling, hoist on her own petard.

At times, just as she seems to be acknowledging some responsibility for unpleasant episodes which have also involved her own behaviour, she turns away, closing down any possibility of a negotiated peace. For example, in her account of her diagnostic consultation, she admits to herself that she is being unjustly hostile to her oncologist, "Onc Doc": "Someone forecasting your death might not be your enemy" (Diski, 2016, p. 3), only to return immediately to the attack. Further, she attributes her slow death from lung cancer to "the wicked cruelty of nature", yet she is pictured on the front cover of her memoir as a younger woman, with cigarette in hand. As opposed to taking all responsibility - or none, as the paradigm of abuser and abused dictates - apportioning degrees of responsibility requires forbearance and balanced judgment. For Diski, it is typically the other and not herself who is at fault. But given that only the contrary would offer her an alternative within her locked-in view, the prospect of a return to the suicidal, wrist-cutting days in a psychiatric hospital of her twenties if it were otherwise, would be very real.

Shame is mentioned in Diski's confession; part of her shame derives from the identity allotted to her by her abusive parents – the replacement of the pretty little girl that she was with an object from a paedophile's fantasy of forbidden love – and part, from what she has in her imagination and in reality, done both to herself and others. Emotions researcher Thomas Scheff claims that shame denotes a crisis feeling of intense disgrace which, if it threatens, most of us try to repress. If that is impossible, we try to re-label the feeling as something that can happen to anyone – perhaps, as Diski calls it, mere "embarrassment" (Scheff, 2015, p. 112). A study carried out by Elias argued that between 1500 and 1900, 'shaming' became centrally important in the socialisation of children by their parents and teachers, while simultaneously, the actual experience of being shamed was gradually less spelt out. Increasingly, feelings of shame and episodes of having been shamed were repressed; "it had become taboo" to mention it (as cited in Scheff, 2015, p. 115).

Scheff also refers to a study by Helen Lewis, a psychoanalyst who researched feelings emerging in psychotherapy sessions. Among the patterns of behaviour that she noted was one she called "bypassed shame", in which a jab of feeling ashamed would typically be followed first by obsessive and rapid thought and then, by imaginary replays of the offending scene in order for the subject to devise a more telling response (Scheff, 2015, p. 117). This account aptly describes Diski's experience in the diagnostic interview; her first response is a flood of embarrassment – or shame – held at bay by "obsessive and rapid thought". Then follows a spate of fantasies, in which Diski mentally reverses the humiliating arrangement and in various scenarios, becomes the sadistic ringmaster, with "Onc Doc" as the victim; she regains control by envisaging the required telling response. Shame is a very primitive emotion, usually related to infants' experiences of feeling repugnant to their caretakers. Perhaps Diski's parents had attributed 'bad behaviour' like initiating sexual games to her, rather than accepting the responsibility for it themselves.

Diski: Ingratitude: Summary

Diski appears to have unconsciously believed that the diagnosis of terminal cancer was thought by the oncologist and his assistant to represent something utterly unacceptable about her. Having always believed that she carried a fatal flaw – something unidentifiable to her but intuited by others – she was convinced that dying would deliver her to a monstrous destiny, to where "the terror squats, rat or raptor, its razor-sharp claws digging into that interior organ where all dreaded things ... live in me" (Diski, p. 143). It is otherwise difficult to explain her reaction of engulfing shame to the diagnosis, followed by a sustained wish to punish the doctor for his presumed attack on her. Arguably, given that her parents had apparently no families with children as friends, and neither understanding of the nature of childhood nor a capacity for empathy, Diski would probably have had repeated experiences as an infant of being at one moment unwanted – even repugnant if she had used her nappy – and the next, adorably sexy, but never just a regular little girl. Accordingly, Diski could develop few confident counter-intuitions to balance her damaging certainties about herself and others. And arguably, with so little positive input to her sense of intrinsic value, Diski never possessed the kind of self-esteem that can survive experiences capable of undermining it.

Unfortunately, she experienced her oncologist as distant, as avoiding personal contact with her about her cancer; had he been able to provide a more open and direct interaction with her, it might have eased her embarrassment – or shame – about feeling somehow very bad and dirty inside, rather than the tragically dying human being she actually was. Having to face death in such an irremediable condition leaves Diski in a parlous state.

Gould: I regret nothing

Gould is not particularly introspective, but he is aware of his faults, and of how others might see him. Addressing the disclosures he has made in his memoir, he first acknowledges being insufficiently sympathetic to his loved ones since he developed cancer and began writing his memoir; he explains that he has been responding to an irresistible sense of purpose that has driven him on. In addition, he does accept as reasonable the criticism that what he says in his memoir crosses certain lines in the sand, and concedes that he has gone further than some people might think was well-judged. Moreover, he is aware that there are people who might even say that he should not have written some of the things that he has in fact written.

In response to his critics, Gould points out that those people who are most important to him have seen what he wrote. Gail has read everything he has written, as have his daughters, Georgia and Grace. But he wants it to be clear that he alone, and no one else, has decided what will be included in his memoir, and furthermore, he is quite aware that in doing so, at times he demonstrates quite some egotism, and an absence of humility.

On the other hand, many people have told him to be honest – including a number of doctors and surgeons – and in particular, to give a true account of the surgery he underwent. So he feels that he has done what is right. And although he accepts that he should perhaps have been more restrained, he did take care to be fair in what he had to say. Having said all that, however, he would not hesitate to do it again, because in his opinion, the benefits have been immense. For example, Gail has certainly benefited from it. Having once been reserved about cancer and death, she now wants to be more open about it, and is actually insisting that more information should be made available to the public.

In this confessional passage, Gould can be pictured as the charismatic leader who orchestrated the election campaigns to victory of UK Labour Prime Minister, Tony Blair. He knows that he is opinionated and arrogant, and evidently believes that in his public life – coupled with his shrewdness and ability to manipulate people's emotions – his self-confidence is an asset which he should keep in play. But it is less acceptable to him that on occasion, he treats his family in a similar way; he knows that sometimes they disagree with his tactics, and that he has often taken no notice of their opinions.

Only his negative revelations about his first surgery seem to give Gould pause; he feels the need to justify himself by quoting the medical fraternity's support for his disclosures about the first surgeon who, having been insufficiently radical in his surgical approach, may have contributed to the prematurity of Gould's death. Having acknowledged earlier that he was also culpable for agreeing to the surgery, however, he feels that it is his duty to 'go public', and inform others who may be similarly in jeopardy, and liable to make negative choices.

Gould: I regret nothing: Summary

In contrast with Diski, Gould is self-confident and sure of the value of what he has to offer; at times, there is an evangelical quality to his project of informing and saving others by his example. There is also an ingenuous spontaneity and warm-heartedness about him which is disarming – and no doubt allows him to get away with a good deal – but he is committed to his memoir and to his mission, and can be trusted to see them through.

Taylor: Missing Mum

Thinking back to her brain surgery almost a year ago reminds Taylor of her mother, whom she still misses so much. When she received the diagnosis of the brain tumour, she was offered a choice between surgical intervention to cut it out, or radiotherapy to reduce it. Either one would be effective, but each involved its own risks. She lay awake in bed, talking over the alternatives in her head with Mum, comforted by feeling that her thoughts were being listened to as attentively as if Mum were still alive. She needed Mum's advice; typically unable to decide on her best course of action, she was sure that Mum would know what she should do. Finally, feeling a longing to be in touch with her that seemed to bring Mum a little closer, she was able to choose the operation, but she confided to Mum as she did so that she was fifty percent persuaded that it would be better if she never woke up. She was sure that Mum would understand this feeling; there was no doubt in her mind that trapped in the institution, Mum would have prayed every night to be released into God's care. Returning to the present, Taylor notes that conjuring up talking to Mum like this makes her feel that she is once more a little girl, and she finds herself longing for some – indeed, any – indication that Mum has not given up on her.

Marriages enjoy varying levels and amounts of communication and for Taylor, it is the Mum within rather than her husband, Shin, to whom she turns for advice in this crisis. It sounds as if Taylor had not told Shin that half-hoping to die during the surgery was on her mind; perhaps she had spared him that. As she lay in bed in a dreamlike state, Taylor's imaginary companion was an earlier version of her mother – the Mum who could always handle a crisis, and who was her all-round childhood heroine – rather than the Mum in an institution for the demented, whom Taylor had deserted. Taken together, the news of the brain tumour and her fears of being disabled by the proposed surgery had apparently caused Taylor to regress, and to feel adrift and motherless and finally, to half hope that she would not survive the operation. Now several years on from that time, Taylor constantly scans her small world for some sign that the Mum who is such an integral part of her is not so disappointed in her that she no longer cares what becomes of her.

Even though they all suffered from major incapacities and repellent symptoms, none of the other participants considered euthanasia to deliver them from the ugliness or distress of becoming cancer-ridden and helpless. Moreover, despite having been terminally ill for so long, Taylor seems to have been as well supported throughout by medical services and her family as any other participant. Arguably, however, while facing a slow disfiguring death could have played a part in her tendency to regress into suicidality, it may not be its fundamental cause. It may rather have been that ten years ago, having just received a terminal diagnosis, Taylor was further traumatised by feeling that in her hour of greatest need, now incapacitated by dementia, her mother was permanently lost to her. Ever since then, she has had to bear the inconsolable loneliness of a child who, having turned away from a broken mother, has felt that, in her turn, she is in danger of abandonment. Early in the piece, she was able to suppress her awareness of this grievous loss, and to write two successful books. Once having become too sick to maintain the façade of business as usual, however, and with death now an imminent rather than a distant reality, she seems to have found the loss of the connection with her mother painfully distressing.

Taylor: Missing Mum: Summary

At this stage, Taylor still has little confidence in her ability to exist independently – forever separate from Mum – and accordingly, she does not yet feel able to manage the last months of her life without her mother's support.

Confessions: Summary

While Gould's confession reveals issues which are eventually resolved, Diski's and Taylor's remain recalcitrant.

How dying is prepared for

Substantive contributions are made by all participants to this sub-category, although by now much weakened by his illness, Hitchens' entries are often very brief. The task facing them now is to find a steadying and authentic basis from which to let life go, and accept death.

How it ends for each participant

Diski

Having to give in and embrace a platitude, Diski reluctantly acknowledges that her life is a journey that is ending: "Much as I hate it, the journey – that … metaphor – keeps popping into my head … From the slap of being told that it's incurable to a sort of acceptance of the upcoming end" (Diski, p. 148). By now faced with an unavoidable submission to dying, she expresses her profound disappointment that her life has not fulfilled its earlier promise:

> [Y]ou realise that it is about time … for the forward journey. There must have been hope at the start, thoughts of something exciting or eventful, and now it's time to be going home … An adventure the other way.
>
> (Diski, p. 246)

She is also afraid of the physical act of dying, due to the presence of both cancer and terminal pulmonary fibrosis in her lungs:

> I will be fighting for breath with both [diseases] … although the … nurse calmed my fears by explaining the steps they take … so that I …

> die unconscious and in some comfort with the aid of intravenous … drugs.
>
> (Diski, p. 154)

Moreover, her Advance Care Plan for dying safely may have collapsed:

> I no longer trust the hospice key worker's assurance that the dying process can be made painless … [The hospice] … couldn't possibly guarantee … a room for me when the time came for dying … I was shaken and distressed.
>
> (Diski, p. 161)

She tries to recover her composure, but she does not sound convinced by her own words: "I'm perfectly sure that there are quiet deaths that creep up on you gently … thanks to skilful palliative care, and that I must hope for that sort of ending" (Diski, p. 167). She finds some brief consolation in being part of the many gone before: "That little cancer in my lung … will kill me, but something would have … [N]ot to speak to me … of 'bravery'. I need to be told … of the millions who've died already" (Diski, p. 209). At times, she even finds a giddy thrill in the prospect of dying:

> Where am I going? Nobody knows … There is a kind of excitement. This, that I've never done … an absolute otherness, nothingness, knowinglessness. That everyone has done, will do … [T]he world going on… without me … My turn.
>
> (Diski, p. 211)

Fundamentally, however, her fear of dying remains undiminished: "And the terror. I'm … seeing a counsellor once a week who has spent ten years … getting people ready for death" (Diski, p. 211). Finally, her sense of having always been marked out for calamity resurfaces:

> There's only one piece of magic left if faith is left out. Love, there's love. But if I arrived on earth without a capacity for faith … with a death sentence tattooed on me.… how the hell [can I] … trust in love?
>
> (Diski, p. 207)

Nearing the end of the memoir, she feels that she has never belonged in this life which, as it ends, has from its very beginning been destined to be erased by its infinite replacements over time:

> Not living in my place … As one might sit on the edge of a chair that is waiting for another occupant … [A] ticking of a clock that will go on ticking after you leave and after the next occupant too.
>
> (Diski, p. 246)

Believing herself destined by fate to be an alien and alienated being, Diski expects to face a correspondingly martyred death.

Gould

Preparing for his death two years after the original cancer diagnosis, Gould's experience could not be more different from the ordeal suffered by Diski. Ensconced in the driver's seat, he believes that there are advantages in his having this foreknowledge of his early death; it is allowing him to reconstruct time, to use it so that it serves his needs. Looking back, he remembers having no sense of purpose when he first realised that an early death was probably in the offing, but he very soon formulated a purpose – to find a purpose. After that, he seems to have intuitively known what he wanted to do in the time left to him. First, he invites his two daughters to join him on a wonderful journey to those places from his past which were most meaningful to him, places where he used to spend time as a boy. As they went from one place to another, they became more and more infused with joy. Gould is certain that this could only happen because his daughters know, as he does, that he is going to die soon, and that sharing this awareness allowed them all to give themselves up completely to this difficult, and potentially distressing expedition.

Next, he chooses a burial plot in the famous Highgate Cemetery, from which his transition after death will take place; once there, he expresses pleasant surprise that this world of the dead is not as he had anticipated. Looking round him, he can see that instead, it is the right place for him to come in order to become something different, since this is what happens at death. And it will be something else, too, something that is good for life; having obtained a bigger plot for the purpose, he intends it to be a communal meeting spot, a venue for family and friends to meet in remembrance of him, and to enjoy each other's company. Altogether, he is profoundly satisfied; he feels that knowing that this is where he will spend eternity is an enormous stride forward, and it gives him immense comfort to know he will be there.

A Christian believer, he predicts that death will be transfiguring; he imagines that dying will be difficult, but its ultimate outcome will be sublime. And although he would have to accept it for his family's sake if he were offered the opportunity to go on living, he does not himself wish to do so. It is his greatest wish to be just where he is now, and to die in his present state of mind, a quite other, and a finer person than he used to be. Feeling at the peak of his development as a person, Gould is convinced that this is the exquisitely right time for him to die.

Hitchens

An antitheist, Hitchens has no expectation of an afterlife; his attention is entirely taken up with the earthly life that remains. In fact, he is the only participant who, even before his terminal illness, wanted to be present at his final moments. In order to experience death and not just undergo it, he wants to be completely conscious as he dies; if an event belongs to his life on this earth, he wants to be there for it. In that connection, since he will have ample opportunity in the time ahead to be dead to the world, he feels that taking sleeping draughts at this stage is just throwing his life away.

Rather than some distance away in the future, his death is now imminent, and he finds that he is giving a good deal of thought to it; in doing so, he notices how much more even than usual, he is operating in two minds. On the one hand, he is trying to prepare himself to die with fortitude, but on the other, he is as focused as ever on how to stay alive. Accordingly, no matter what the illness hurls in his direction, he remains determined to fight it. But he is also only too aware that life is fast running out; his inexorable downhill slide has been made even steeper by the hospital recently landing him with a nasty staph pneumonia that almost killed him. Ever since then, he has been overcome by an engulfing lethargy and weariness, in which he can already detect the toxic seeds of his impending surrender.

Soon after he wrote these entries, Hitchens was reduced by his weakness to recording only brief jottings; nonetheless, he kept his journal until he died.

Mayne

Like Gould, Mayne was given his terminal diagnosis after two years of frequently brutal treatment for his cancer and poignantly, soon after having been given the all-clear; his response is contained in a short postscript to his memoir, which begins:

> The cancer has returned, and the options now are limited. This doesn't change anything I have written ... I have had the ... privilege of [reviewing] ... my life: of learning more about its meaning, about myself and about those I love.
>
> (Mayne, p. 243)

The suffering caused by the resurgent cancer is harrowing; he describes it graphically:

> The hardest thing ... is to accept an unpleasant open wound in the throat which ... possesses the worst scent in the world, the smell of cancer ... [But] I find myself saying: 'I can do all things through Christ who strengthens me'.
>
> (Mayne, pp. 248–249)

His prognosis – survival for only a few more months – is also daunting: "There is ... shock in hearing it spelled out so finally, and part of me ... feels nothing but fear and dismay. And with A., [his wife, Alison] I am [sometimes] ... wracked by sobs" (Mayne, p. 250). However, they have come to a decision; he will accept no further chemotherapy: "I don't intend to spin things out. What lies ahead ... contains times best kept private ... [T]hese last days [are about] ... not the *amount* of time left to me but its *quality*" (Mayne, p. 246). Resolute, he feels well-sustained: "I go into ... my final weeks or months knowing that I don't go alone, but supported by family and friends and ... three religious communities" (Mayne, p. 244). He is satisfied with the legacy of his memoir:

> [I have appreciated] the discipline (and therapy) of writing ... [B]ooks are about ... what matters to us most, our desire to 'speak what we feel, not what we ought to say' ... [A] small – and sometimes quite risky – act of love.
>
> (Mayne, pp. 245–246)

By now, he is secure in his relationship with God: "In the evening I simply make a final act of committal of myself and my loved ones ... 'Father ... Into your hands I commend my spirit ... O Lord God of truth'" (Mayne, p. 249). Finally, observing that we each choose to die in our own way, he counsels: "[We can try] ... to unseal our clenched fists and let go of what we have been given with open hands. To die with gratitude ... is the greatest gift we can leave those who love us" (Mayne, pp. 250–251). Like Gould, Mayne is ready to die, though unlike Gould, he is anguished about leaving those he loves so soon. Indeed, he is a prime example of how it is possible to feel fear and sorrow about the forthcoming parting and yet, able to accept death with grace.

Taylor

Unlike the other participants, Taylor has been terminally ill for ten years; her initial response to the diagnosis – exemplifying creative disregard – was a desire to seize the moment, and to produce a piece of work that was authentically hers. She describes her reaction when she held her first novel in her hand; she had a feeling of incomparable joy, and the thought that now, she could die happy. More recently, dying has prompted her to look back over her life, and in this last book, her memoir, she seeks to uncover the sequences and moments of decision that represented watershed moments for her over the years. Regretting that she had nothing recorded by her mother which might have guided her understanding of how she had experienced her life, Taylor wants to leave an account of her own life for her sons to read, and to muse over after her death. A service they provide to the dying, her home nursing service volunteer has also recorded her story and put it into a book for the family; she appreciates this, but wants to add a more personal volume, a narrative of her own creation.

Attributing it to having lived both in Queensland and abroad, Taylor finds herself unable to identify somewhere that feels like home for a final resting place. Poignantly, she reflects that she can never hope to have a genuine sense of belonging, and must do without it. As a result, it is not obvious where her ashes should be spread; there is some discussion about this going on in the family, but Taylor herself feels that quite candidly, she is not too bothered about what becomes of her after death. Now, Taylor's confession as her death approaches that she lacks all sense of belonging is no less affecting than Diski's, but the self-disparaging quality of the comments about not being too bothered that follow is striking. As previously observed, Taylor cannot readily resolve painfully conflicted feelings and at times, as she does here, she switches to a brusque statement, in which the recently suppressed feelings are still unrelatedly present in her use of language. The bleakness of having no home, no receptive place to lie for eternity, remains in her reference to not caring what becomes of her, as well as in her next statement, in which as seen earlier, she refers to asking her husband to decorate an urn for her ashes, and when he is ready, to just "toss me out". Taylor appears not to notice this tendency to rough talk, or how she dissociates her attitudes from their emotionally-affecting origins. In addition, as noted earlier in the chapter, in *Taylor: To be or not to be,* she regularly finds herself trapped in two minds, unable to resolve their conflicting standpoints. In this case, she expresses herself both as thoughtful adult, and as homeless waif – on the one hand, as one who, with her family, is making all the appropriate arrangements for her forthcoming death, but on the other, as one whose passing will not matter to anyone, especially herself.

Taylor's tendency to become caught on the horns of various dilemmas seems to be related to her preoccupations regarding her mother, to her fundamental conflict as to whether she and her mother were, and still are, happily at one, or unhappily torn apart. Until now, Taylor has not been able to separate from her mother and move forward with her own life and death. Indeed, the opportunity to move forward into an independent life and a peaceful death has so far seemed out of the question for Taylor. And yet, as it turns out, with the help of her creative and protective unconscious mind, Taylor does find a way through her dilemma. Somehow putting aside the brooding about mistreating her mother, she begins this last narrative thinking about what matters to her in the present – her own family – and about losing them when she dies.

She is aware that when death comes, there is much that she will miss; first and foremost, the presence in her life of Shin, her husband for these last thirty-one years, closely followed by the beloved faces of her adult sons, Nat and Dan. Going beyond her immediate circle, she feels keenly the pain of parting with the world and everything in it, and the sense of a future in which she could take it for granted that she would be around to see how things turn out. In a way unique among the participants, she experiences her life as very slowly fading away; her world has dwindled to two rooms, and much as a child might, she just lies on her couch and daydreams. She is aware that her life is coming to a close; she is finding that these days, far from stirring her into wakefulness, the sound of early morning birdsong outside her room fills her with longing to drift back into the oblivion from which she came. For Taylor, as for Gould, there is a kind of happiness and peace in dying. Both participants are living entirely in the moment; for Gould, it is intense and ecstatic, full of life and movement, while for Taylor, it is dreamy and abstracted. She feels gently carried along – unresisting and at times barely conscious – towards a longed-for state of union with her mother, and from there, with everything that is, or ever was. Taylor had no religion; her longing to drift into a kind of oceanic oblivion has a pantheistic quality.

Even though she steadily became weaker and continued keep the euthanasia drug in reserve, Taylor eventually stopped actively planning to use it, or even to think about it. According to this last stage of her account, she appears to be slipping away into a merciful oblivion; it seems likely that this relatively gentle dying was one reason for her finally withdrawing from the need to euthanise herself. And perhaps the attentive care she received from her husband allowed her to imagine, in her regressed state, that her mother was there to love and protect her; certainly, she seems to have known instinctively that it was at last safe for her to allow herself to give in, and let go. If this is right, a dying person imagining themselves in a happy dreamworld may, most appropriately, be spared any attempts to draw them back to everyday reality.

How it ends for each participant: Issues arising

For Diski and Hitchens, the time has come to disengage and withdraw. Having tried to achieve "a sort of" acceptance of her imminent death, Diski has recently been let down by the local hospice over a promise to make her death bearable. In anguish, she asks: How she can believe in salvation by faith or love? Trapped by, rather than ready for her imminent death, in profound disappointment, she is beginning to withdraw into herself. Also emotionally distant, Hitchens writes as if meta-reporting on how he is handling his situation. He underplays the emotional aspect of his rapid decline, and requires his companions to do the same; take, for example, his last observation, that he has been overcome by an engulfing lethargy and weariness, in which he can already detect the seeds of his impending surrender. Such a statement does not invite comment: only chiming in with something like: "What a bugger!" seems a possible conversational move. Having previously considered vetoing would-be empathic advances from visitors, Hitchens has found that communicating in unequivocal statements which present no entry points, is an effective technique for keeping would-be sympathisers at arm's length.

Now close to death, Gould, Mayne, Taylor and Diski are all preoccupied with issues regarding quality of the life that remains. Although he is not the only participant to think that he would reject more life if it were on offer, Gould is singular in his conviction that because he knows that he is dying, the quality of his life has reached its peak and therefore, that this is the right time for him to die. Mayne's Christianity is more down-to-earth than Gould's; it is intellectual and spiritual rather than mystical. By now, his anguish about God's seeming remoteness has gone, and his most profound conflicts have been resolved; these insights sustain him throughout his trials. At this point he refuses further chemotherapy, favouring quality of time over its amount. Often inconsistent, Taylor at times seems to believe herself to be ultimately dispensable and yet, like Gould and Mayne, she also feels that she has had a fortunate life; she observes that she would be happy to know that her children have been as fortunate as she has. She never has to make use of her euthanasia drug or her troubling Advance Care Plan; when her time comes, she is ready to go peacefully. While pondering whether or not to take the final offer of vomit-inducing pills, like Mayne, Diski has considered the question of quality versus quantity of the time ahead. Arguably however, Gould and Mayne do not mean the same thing by "quality time" as Diski does. For his part, Gould is set to die a happy, even ecstatic man. And when Mayne suggests that we can die with gratitude for the lives we have been given, he has much to be grateful for; he has enjoyed the most rewarding of experiences with work, friends and family, and has been recognised with a knighthood. A modest man, he nonetheless knows his own value. By contrast, despite her status as a Fellow of the Royal Society of Literature, her library of admired publications, and numbering many famous and talented people among her friends, a dying Diski feels that neither she nor her life has amounted to much. Arguably, when she considers quality of life over quantity, for Diski – who seemingly cannot value anything that is hers – it is not to achieve the best, only to avoid the worst. For her, living with cancer and with death in the offing is bad, but vomiting all the way there would render it intolerable.

All the participants are involved in imagining how they will face up to the end and here, there is an unanticipated finding. For the atheists, weak or unsuccessful aspects of the self are to be disowned; Taylor abandons her now disposable body-self, Hitchens has banned all self-pity or need for sympathy, while in despair, Diski sees nothing much in herself or her life that is worth preserving. By contrast, believers Mayne and Gould face death feeling no need for preparatory grooming; in the words of Charlotte Elliott's 1835 hymn, they approach death-as-transition:

"Just as I am without one plea … that Thou bidst me come to Thee". (Retrieved from https://en.wikipedia.org/wiki/Just_As_I_Am(hymn))

How it ends for each participant: Summary

The participants are preoccupied with reviewing what they have experienced so far and what lies ahead. A fear of vulnerability to loss of control from experiencing more emotional pain than they can handle, has led Diski and Hitchens to disengage and withdraw. As seen in Chapter 5, they also reacted to the shock of the initial cancer diagnosis with distancing and avoidance. For these two participants, disengagement appears to have become their instinctive response to the threat of sustained emotional stress.

Now in their final months of life, Gould, Mayne, Taylor and Diski are all preoccupied in different ways with issues about quality of life. Gould believes that his quality of life has reached its zenith and that now is the right time for him to die. Despite being gravely ill, Mayne's relationship with God sustains him as he moves towards death. At this point, favouring quality of time over quantity, he refuses further chemotherapy; he can die with gratitude for the good life that he has had. Taylor longs to feel that the mother within still loves her and at last, seems to imagine that she does; she is being carried along on a tide of birdsong toward a kind of pantheistic oblivion. For Diski, a life that may seem rewarding to others is of little value to her; feeling that her life is infinitely replaceable with those who will follow her, she cannot identify, and so feel that she has fulfilled, a unique purpose of her own.

Finally, the study suggests that where dying individuals like Mayne and Gould understand perfection to exist in an external deity, they are unconcerned about their flaws, and look forward to spending eternity with a welcoming God. By contrast, a non-believer like Diski is convinced that she has no value beyond death or, like the earlier Taylor, that after death and cremation, what remains of her can just be tossed out. Hitchens does not negate his value, but he does not want to die in a vulnerable state; he wants to be strong, stoical and independent, to put his best foot forward at the end. The possible significance of the contrast between these two groups is discussed further in Chapter 8, *Themes in the experience of dying*.

Disposing of one's earthly remains

Gould and Taylor both refer to the need for a final resting place; Gould is focused on choosing the right plot in which to spend eternity, while by contrast, Taylor decides that her family can spread her ashes wherever they wish. Research online shows that Mayne's ashes were buried alongside his peers in Westminster Abbey. (*Westminster Abbey Guide for Visitors*. Retrieved from http://www.westminsterabbey.org/ourhistory/people/michael-mayne)

Similarly, investigation online revealed that Hitchens donated his body to medical research (*Find a grave*. Retrieved 7/05/18, from https://www.findagrave.com/memorial/82028325/christopher-eric-hitchens)

How Diski's body was disposed of is not known, though she once said that she favoured cremation over burial.

For Gould and Mayne, the choice of final resting place was meaningful, while neither Hitchens nor Taylor certainly, nor Diski probably, had any interest in it at all. It might seem that this suggests that Christians care about disposal rituals while the irreligious do not; in fact, however, this does not seem be the case. Although Gould chose his own grave plot, Mayne's burial-place was prescribed, and he expressed no further interest in it in his memoir. Now, it might be thought that, in our secular society, we are too rationalistic to be concerned about what happens to our bodies after death, but if that were the case, organ donation would perhaps be more common than it is.

Arguably then, when people die a protracted and painful death – often characterised by pain, disfigurement and loss of vital functions – they withdraw their investment from their bodies, and live in their minds and hearts; the body is finally discarded like a tattered overcoat, and its destination is of little interest to its erstwhile owner. Alone amongst the participants, Gould took considerable trouble over choosing his grave plot in Highgate Cemetery, in London; having done so, he made a YouTube video in which he stood on his grave plot, and talked to the camera about how glad he was to have decided that this was the place where he would spend eternity. His emphasis on the importance of his grave as a meeting-place for friends and family may suggest that, unique amongst the participants, he imagined that his transfigured self might have some kind of benevolent presence on earth.

Disposing of one's earthly remains: Summary

Although Mayne, Gould and Taylor planned their funerals, only Gould took an active interest in bodily disposal. Possibly, ravaged cancer sufferers generally withdraw investment in their bodily selves.

How dying is prepared for: Summary

All the participants wanted to be intimately known and remembered by their families and they all gave them full access to their memoirs and other memorabilia. Hitchens, Gould, Mayne and Taylor made provision for the disposal of their bodies after death, although only Gould took an interest in it. As death approaches and their emotional suffering increases, Diski and Hitchens withdraw and disengage. Arguably, close involvement with others is not what all dying individuals want; although it may be hard for their loved ones to accept, sometimes the dying need to withdraw into themselves, and to leave practical arrangements – planning funerals, for example – to the family. Certainly, religiously-based, observant cultures apart, posthumous obsequies may not be so much for the dying, as for those they leave behind.

Four participants – Diski, Gould, Mayne and Taylor – are involved in making decisions concerning quality time. For Gould, Mayne and Taylor, quality time entails being free to live under the best conditions available to them, and to die without vexatious life-prolonging treatment. By contrast, Diski's choice hovers between a life sustained by medication but with no quality, and a medication-free, but probably earlier death for which she feels totally unready; for his part, Hitchens has always wanted more life and accordingly, to remain combative, he has accepted all medication to the end. Although no conclusions can be drawn from such a small sample, it is noticeable that choices about prioritising best quality time are specific to the three participants who remain engaged with others. Further, even this small study shows that due to their individual ways of interacting with the illness experience, significant differences exist amongst the participants about what constitutes quality time, and why and when it is time to let go. Accordingly, it does not support the idea of providing one-size-fits-all versions of Advance Care Planning formats even to the terminally-ill, let alone the still well.

Finally, the study suggests that, where dying individuals understand perfection to exist in an external deity and a welcome to await them in heaven, they seem unconcerned about their earthly flaws; by contrast, non-believers judge themselves robustly or even harshly, and some may even impose a self-improvement regimen on themselves as death approaches. Given that the number of participants in this study is small, no conclusion can be drawn from this; however, further investigation would almost certainly be rewarding.

Part II. Final thoughts

The last words of each memoir follow.

Diski

As it is enigmatic, Diski's final entry is contextualised by inserting the first six words of the theme which her last words conclude. As her memoir draws to a close, she is preoccupied with thoughts about her mother, whose mental disturbance so damaged her attempts to introduce her fatherless daughter to the family's Jewish traditions. In the memoir's final paragraph, Diski is recalling her mother's attitude when she first began to menstruate, or as her mother called it, 'being unwell', and her way of introducing her daughter to traditional cleansing rituals:

> She would have to slap my face when it first started ... so appalled and panicked was she. All that, I learned [later] ... was part of Jewish tradition ... very hard to separate from the mad rituals of my mother.
>
> (Diski, p. 249)

In her final words, she tries to continue with this theme, but completely loses the thread:

> Unwell, after all, is not ill ... The mishmash suddenly made the only sense, mishmash whirled around and pulled together in a kind of Disney dance, which hasn't been made, but should have been because it is a much better story than *Beauty and the Beast.*
>
> (Diski, p. 250)

It is impossible to know what Diski intends by these final words; her ability to think coherently seems to have given way under the stress of dying. Indeed, when understood as a fear of falling apart while still alive, Diski's intuition that dying will bring on a state of breakdown has turned out to be prescient. And yet, perhaps this collapse is also self-protective, a refuge she has unconsciously found from her recent coherent, but intolerably tormenting thoughts. Perhaps in an unconscious attempt to care for herself, the capacity for unconditional love that she feels for her grandchildren may have at last been extended to include herself. Arguably, as discussed in the previous Sub-set: *Resolution of conflicts*, such a development could even amount to a kind of redemption. With no explanation, her memoir breaks off here, some weeks before she died; it seems likely that she could no longer write for publication.

Gould

Written shortly before his death from an antibiotic-resistant infection, Gould's final entry is typically upbeat: "I am approaching the door marked Death. What lies beyond it may be the worst of things. But I believe it will be the best of things" (Gould, p. 143).

Hitchens

Hitchens had also developed an incurable pneumonia infection, and for some time, had been recording only jottings. Written the night he died, Hitchens' farewell message is unusually long; it appears to have been profoundly meaningful to him. A quotation from Alan Lightman's novel, *Einstein's dreams* (Lightman, 1993, p. 121), it reads:

> With infinite life comes an infinite list of relatives. Grandparents never die, nor do great-grandparents, great-aunts … [Hitchens' ellipsis points] and so on, back through the generations, all alive and offering advice. Sons never escape from the shadows of their fathers. Nor do daughters of their mothers. *No one ever comes into his own* … [Hitchens' emphasis and ellipsis points]. Such is the cost of immortality. No person is whole. No person is free.
>
> (Hitchens, pp. 92–93)

Unlike the other participants, Hitchens had never before recorded any reason to accept death. In fact, his death was not yet expected by the hospital staff, but knowing how close he was to surrender, Hitchens himself probably realised that it was imminent. Independence of mind was precious to him; now on the brink of death, it dawned on him that our mortality is the price that we have to pay to secure it.

Mayne

Closing his memoir some weeks before his death, Mayne's love of watching the changing seasons, and his philosophy of the cyclical nature of life and death come together to make this homage to the grand scheme of things his farewell to his readers:

> In these past weeks I have been pondering on the ordered rhythm of the seasons ... Each witness to change, to the annual pattern of death and new life. Each summons us to a sense of wonder at nature's *cantus firmus*. A melody that is both hopeful and enduring.
>
> (Mayne, p. 251)

Taylor

Taylor's final words are written as a screenplay; screenwriting had been her profession before she was diagnosed with cancer:

> If I were writing my death scene for a film, my very last moments would go something like this. A montage. Shaky, over-exposed home movie footage of a girl with a dog in dappled sunshine ... arm in arm with her mother in some outback moonscape, crossing the tarmac at an airport with a silver jet in the background. The jet takes off ...
>
> Fade to black.
>
> (Taylor, 2016, p. 147)

The narrative places a modern jet in the background, but the home-movie atmosphere suggests a family scene from long ago. Rather as Gould had it, everything significant exists at once in Taylor's Death Zone; she is a girl again, travelling by jet with her adored mother. In the merging of imagination and reality in Taylor's mind during her dying weeks, the early relationship with her mother has been restored. They embark, forever linked, on a trip to a timeless realm. Her current family is not present; they belong to an ongoing life in which very soon, she will no longer have a place.

Final thoughts: Summary

Gould and Hitchens continued to write their memoirs until they died while Diski, Mayne and Taylor stopped writing some weeks beforehand. There is a tone of finality in the last words of Taylor and Mayne while for Diski, a slip into incoherence is followed by silence.

The two female participants focus at the end on their relationships with their mothers – Diski, to instance the ways in which her mother had failed her, particularly in rendering her disconnected from her Jewish origins, while Taylor, by contrast, sketches a return to her roots and her beloved and protective mother. The final words of the three male participants were not addressed to a person; instead, they each presented the philosophy which expressed their sense of a life experience completed and understood. For Gould, the distillate of his life's experience was: *The times ahead will be the best of times*; for Hitchens: *Our mortality sets us free*, and for Mayne: *Our wonderful God-given world order turns on an eternal cycle of death and new life.* None of these principles thought to govern life and death is new, but for each of these three participants, finally coming to understand what made cosmic sense to him has had to be his own discovery.

In fact, no participant sought to be told what to believe. Evidently, this is something that when our time comes, we have to come to in our own way.

Represented in the final words of these five participants are two very different ways of accepting death. For the women, it seemed natural to turn inwards, to examine and reconstruct their memories and finally, to be drawn towards their origins and in particular, to the relationship with the mother. Unfortunately, for Diski, unlike Taylor, there was no beloved mother within to offer her a refuge, but she may at least have stumbled on an unconscious pathway to closing down her persecuting inner voices. For the men, a principle or a philosophy seemed to represent a steadying base from which they could let go of life. While this sample is too small to generalise to a finding about gender predisposition, it is reasonable to infer that both of these realms can offer an anchorage from which to accept one's death.

Some issues related to gender emerging from the summary of the three data analysis narrative chapters

There were three issues in the data analysis narrative in which the participants were divided according to gender. Firstly, it emerged in Chapter 6, that, concerning attitudes to doctors and medical professionals, the male participants accepted having to endure often brutal treatments carried out without reference to their feelings; their focus was on the effectiveness of the treatment. By contrast, the women looked for a supportive relationship with their treating personnel, but often felt that instead, they were being 'managed', with no concern for their feelings, or even for their personal well-being.

Secondly, as emerged in Chapter 5, regarding their reasons for writing the memoir, the men emphasised the aspects of their memoirs that represented a kind of mission statement; by contrast, Diski and Taylor used their memoirs mainly for more introspective pursuits, such as retrieving and analysing significant relationships.

Thirdly, emerging from the current chapter, Chapter 7, and concerning the final thoughts of their memoirs, the women remained absorbed in their memories of past relationships and at the last, felt drawn towards their origins – especially to their mothers – while for the men, a personal philosophy or a belief system seems to have offered a stable position from which to face death. Now, this investigation is too small to support generalisations about gender or any other predispositions in preparing for death. However, the consistency in direction of their attention by the men as compared with the women across the three sets of findings outlined above, does suggest that in the final crisis of facing death, women feel drawn toward the subjective, to exploring their roots, and their feelings and relationships with those who were significant to them, while men turn outward to the objective and the philosophical, seeking to epitomise a world in which our mortality can be seen to represent the culmination of a life well-lived.

On one point, however, the participants were united throughout the study; it is essential for those who can do so to work with whatever is important to them, and to avoid becoming submerged in their illness; all participants found that their writing provided a creative and restorative balance to the depersonalising ravages of the cancer and its treatment.

Next follows Chapter 8: *Themes in the experience of dying,* which discusses the results of the data analysis in relation to the rest of the book and to the literature, and suggests ways in which the experience of dying in our society might be further humanised and enriched.

References

Diski, J. (2016). *In gratitude*. London and New York: Bloomsbury Publishing.

Gould, P. (2013). *When I die: Lessons from the death zone*. London, UK: Abacus, Little, Brown Book Group.

Hitchens, C. E. (2012). *Mortality*. New York, Boston, MA: Twelve Books.

Mayne, M. C. O. (2006). *The enduring melody*. London: Darton, Longman and Todd.

Scheff, T. (2015). Toward defining basic emotions. *Qualitative Inquiry, 21*(2), 111–121. doi: 10.1177/1077800414550462

Taylor, C. (2016). *Dying: A memoir*. Melbourne: Text Publishing.

Torges, C. M., Nolen-Hoeksma, S., & Stewart, A. J. (2008). Regret resolution, aging, and adapting to loss. *Psychology and Aging, 23*(1), 169–180. doi: 10.1037/0882-7974.23.1.169

8 Themes in the experience of dying

Introduction

Entitled *Reacting to the news: Diagnosis, Living with dying*, and *Acceptance* respectively, the three previous chapters recounted the participants' journey from diagnosis to near-death. To carry the narratives of the participants forward, and to identify which of their experiences were idiosyncratic and which were shared, a chronological presentation of the data was most effective. In the forthcoming chapter, on the other hand, in order to make the best use of the data to enhance our understanding of the broader issues surrounding death and dying, it has to be reorganised into a different format. To facilitate the discussion of commonalities and differences in the participants' experience, and to relate these to recommendations for care of the dying, the data categories have been reorganised into thirty-two inter-connected items or themes and then, further refined, into eleven groups, or clusters of themes.

These findings are examined in the chapter which follows; combining this analysis with appropriate references to the literature, recommendations can be made regarding contemporary society's understanding and management of death and dying. Note that the order in which these data are discussed is geared to the use of the same set of data in Chapter 9, *Conclusions*; that is, it is organised in readiness for the two 'burning questions' which originally motivated the research to be answered.

The chapter is divided into four parts: Part I examines the data relating to the first of the 'burning questions', which asks what it is like to face death, while the data discussed in Part II relates to the second question, which asks how, when we are apparently programmed to seek survival at all costs, we can ever genuinely accept death. Part III gives some accounts of creatively conceived *ars moriendi*, or examples of the art of dying well, while Part IV acknowledges the limitations of the research, and suggests areas which would benefit from further investigation.

Part I. Themes related to what is it like to face death

Part II. Themes related to whether we can become ready to relinquish life and accept death

Part III. *Ars moriendi*: The art of dying well

DOI: 10.4324/9781003392088-8

Part IV. Limitations of the research, and areas for further investigation

Part I. Themes relating to study question 1. What is it like to face death?

First cluster: Participants' reaction to the initial diagnosis

This cluster is made up of three themes.

Theme (i) Attribution of responsibility for contracting cancer

While only four participants considered the question "Why me?", all five participants had an opinion about where the responsibility for contracting cancer lay. For Hitchens, Gould and Taylor, the responsibility was theirs. For Gould and Hitchens, it was continuous hard-living – despite warnings and family concern – which had caused them to be vulnerable to contracting cancer. Similarly, Taylor believed that it was her failure to inspect her sunburnt skin carefully enough that had allowed a melanoma to flourish undetected behind her right knee. Now, there is no inevitable, one-to-one direct line between hard-living or neglected sunburn and cancer, but all three participants were as angry with and blaming of themselves as if there were. On the other hand, even though Mayne had previously had two melanomas removed and Diski had been a cigarette smoker, neither held themselves responsible for developing cancer; both took the view that such a calamity can befall anyone.

Given these contrasting responses to contracting the same disease, it is suggested that people identify the source of their cancer in two distinct ways. Diski and Mayne both understood that their cancers were unwelcome products of their own flesh and bodily processes; by contrast, Gould and Hitchens believed the cancer to be the outcome of an alien invasion, a toxic intruder which had slipped past physiological defences weakened by overwork and hard living. Taylor also identified the cancer as a hostile force to be repelled, but her interpretation of the cause was more nuanced: while she saw the cancer as the effect of over-exposure to the sun, it had to have been mediated by her body turning against itself.

Recommendation

During the diagnostic phase, some benefit may accrue from discovering how a patient understands their cancer to have been caused. For example, individuals like Gould and Hitchens, who see the cancer as an invading alien force, may be more able to accept and profit from the most punishing of treatments, because they interpret it as an all-out fight for survival against colonisation by an external enemy. By contrast, individuals like Mayne, Diski and Taylor, who experience the treatment as one side of a fight which is all taking place within themselves may, as in fact they all did, eventually begin to weigh up the felt damage resulting from the treatment against the benefit that it is expected to confer. Even if the penalty is likely to be an earlier death, they may need to be supported in ending a treatment that is experienced as too destructive to their quality of life to be worth continuing.

Theme (ii) Preparedness for death may be linked more to retirement than to literal age

Gould and Hitchens were both close to sixty and still working full-time when the cancer struck; it had occurred while they were still sufficiently in the thick of life and work to believe a terminal diagnosis to be unseasonable and therefore, in need of explanation. On the other hand, Diski at 67 and Mayne at 76, who had retired from regular employment some years previously, certainly found the cancer diagnosis unwelcome, but not untimely. Taylor's experience was atypical of the participant group; diagnosed with cancer some ten years earlier at the age of fifty, she had given up her freelance work as a screenwriter in order to write some long-postponed novels while she still could.

Nursing academic and expert in aged care, Katherine Froggatt, observes that retirement often leads to the loss of people's links to their former social connections as well as to their work roles (Froggatt, 2001, p. 321). It is possible that, like Diski and Mayne, being sidelined from the midst of life and entering a period generally taken to represent its last phase, activates the individual's awareness that, even if some way off, death is the next port of call. By contrast, for those who like Hitchens, Taylor and Gould, are still fully involved in employed work and the general business of living, such an awareness may still be latent.

Recommendation

Healthcare programs which must rely on public awareness of the need to make end of life arrangements – for example, by completing an Advance Care Plan – may benefit from addressing the retired ahead of those still leading busy work and social lives.

Theme (iii) Patterns of emotional response to diagnosis

Receiving the cancer diagnosis left three participants in great distress. Gould felt terrified at first, Mayne was barely able to control his panic for days, while a weeping Taylor, railing at fate, wanted to turn to her mother for comfort, only to find that she had been institutionalised with dementia. For some time, all three were struggling for composure. By contrast, Hitchens and Diski both responded to the diagnosis in a distant, even satirical fashion. Hitchens dismissed the usual "Why me?" cry as of no interest whatsoever to the universe, while Diski described her now cancer-dominated future as one of "preordained banality" (Diski, p. 1). For both Diski and Hitchens, maintaining an avoidant position in the face of calamity seems to have been a well-established way of dealing with emotional crises. In due course, Mayne, Gould and Taylor regained their equilibrium, while Hitchens managed to sustain his phlegmatic attitude to the end. However, although Diski's mask of ennui did not last long away from the diagnostic interview, her accounts of subsequent consultations with her apparently unresponsive oncologist suggest that whenever she met him, the mask was in place. Ultimately, due partly to persistent non-compliance with chemotherapy, Diski died in a state of breakdown two months short of the minimum time she had been given to live.

Recommendation

Given the enigmatic responses of two out of the five participants to receiving the diagnosis, a number of those who most need support may be similarly concealing their feelings and thus, flying under the radar. To distinguish those hiding acute distress from the genuinely self-contained, careful follow-up would be required. While confrontation of distrustful patients like Diski or Hitchens would probably only antagonise them, they may respond co-operatively to consistent kindness and concern. According to British psychoanalyst and hospice consultant, Colin Parkes, being approached in a courteous way generally elicits co-operation from avoidant cancer patients. Parkes et al. emphasise that avoidance is not denial; in fact, since it is usually due to a fear of losing control, showing avoidant patients that they are in charge, and that they are free to switch their feelings on and off at will, may allow them to feel that they can afford to be more open (Parkes et al., 1996, p. 79). According to Parkes, people's ways of coping should be respected and worked with; there is no 'right' response for all (Parkes et al., 1996, p. 97).

Second cluster: The impossibility of conceptualising our own death

This cluster is made up of two themes.

Theme (iv) What the participant thinks death is

As discussed in the Chapter 2, *Death as enigma*: *Part I*, it is impossible to conceptualise one's own death and indeed, none of the participants could do so. While Hitchens did not contribute, four participants did address this issue; Mayne observed that it is not possible to imagine your own death, Taylor offered the conventional view that death is part of the eternal cycle of birth and death, and Gould provided a description of how he experienced life in the "Death Zone". Diski alone had struggled with defining death, only to have to confess a failure to do so that she ascribed to the limits of language. As it turned out, what she really needed to do was to express her feelings less about death, and more about dying.

Recommendation

For some individuals, being unable to identify death's character and power in words may render it the more alarming, because it defies our attempts to classify and subjugate it. For the terminally-ill reflecting on what lies ahead, however, no matter how difficult it is to talk about, it may not be possible just to bypass and ignore the subject. In fact, it may emerge that like Diski, they are afraid of the process of dying rather than of death itself; healthcare professionals offering death counselling may find that a shift in focus to feelings about the dying process is productive.

Theme (v) Experiencing the reality of death in the grief of loved ones

One of the most painful of the participants' experiences was seeing the reality of their fate reflected in the grief and sorrow of their loved ones. Unable to know what her death meant to herself, Diski could feel its impact by mirroring the anguish felt by her husband, by feeling his loss as if it were hers; after a long and close marriage, Mayne and his wife felt that their having become as if of one flesh, was about to be torn apart; Taylor was profoundly grateful that her husband and sons had each other for support, and before losing each other forever, Gould and his wife had reached and maintained a state of intense intimacy. Hitchens could not bear to have his feelings of grief and loss touched, and seemed to shut off attempts either to reach or to confide in him.

Relationships among persons in families where a loved member is dying are likely to be very fluid, and as family members so often feel each other's pain as well as their own, their boundaries can become entangled. Given that patients usually want to spend as much precious time as possible with their partner and family before the final farewell, they may become something of a composite, a 'patient-with-family'.

Recommendation

From the outset, healthcare personnel will need to resist pressures to be involved in the family dynamics and instead, to make sure to remain outside the family enclave, while always focusing on the facilitation of the patient's progress towards as easeful a death as possible. ICU consultant Charlie Corke advises medical professionals that, in his experience, and despite its problems, enabling families to select someone to act as proxy for the patient and emissary for the family is the most containing and effective way to proceed, especially when the patient is dying in ICU (Corke & Hillman, 2018, July 28, ABC radio interview).

Third cluster: Emotional experiences and their management

This cluster is made up of four themes.

Theme (vi) Main areas of emotional stress

Six areas of emotional concern were significant to all participants – having cancer *per se*; the prospect of parting forever from their spouses and families;

the potential loss of control of everything important to them; having the support of family and friends, medical professionals and others; finding the resources in the self and in the community to manage painful feelings and finally, needing to maintain their individuality and, rather than becoming 'unpersons' – 'the terminally ill' or 'advanced cancer patients' – to be recognised as their authentic selves. Showing perseverance and courage in their responses to the consequences of a terminal cancer diagnosis, the participants demonstrated a capacity for wide-ranging emotional work and resourcefulness in accessing the support they needed to do it. Taylor and Diski alone sought professional help from a death counsellor; Taylor was unimpressed by her counsellor, and while Diski did not record the outcome of her consultations, she did not report feeling any benefit from it.

Recommendation

For those who wish to enlist professional help, there are several professional services cited in the literature for reducing the likelihood of depression and anxiety in the terminally ill. Of these, there is one type in particular worthy of consideration if one-to-one counselling is too short-term, does not offer enough support, or puts too much on pressure to 'succeed' in relieving anxiety on the two persons involved. McDermott, Hill and Morgan, a group of Australian psychologists, describe working with a group of advanced breast cancer sufferers to lessen their anxiety and depression, and to improve their quality of life. Despite the regular deaths of its members, the group itself continued to remain alive, to the benefit of the current members. McDermott et al.'s explanation of the effectiveness of the group in supporting its members was that, due to the bonds of intimacy and affection among them, they knew that they would "live on" in the minds of those who had accompanied them to the end; the struggles and achievements that they might not be able to speak so openly about at home would be addressed and remembered within the group (McDermott et al., 2009, p. 174).

Theme (vii) The fear of being abandoned when facing death

Three of the participants expressed a fear of being abandoned by someone on whom they were highly dependent. Having suffered abuse and desertion by her parents from infancy on, and having feared meeting the same fate from her sponsor, Doris Lessing, Diski was in constant terror of abandonment in her last months of life. While she seemed to feel secure with her husband, she was afraid of being denied help from her local hospice staff in her final hours. Moreover, she feared that, in the act of dying, she would be abandoned by the cosmos into eternal exile. Mayne had been abandoned by his suicide father, and for some time, he feared losing touch with God in his final anguish. Taylor was afraid of being abandoned by her greatly loved other, her mother, in retribution for her neglect, and of having to die while still unable to feel her mother's presence within. Mayne and Taylor both recovered their confidence in a benevolent outcome, but Diski remained in despair.

Psychiatrist Mark Sullivan points out that hopelessness is not just an absence of hope, it is an attachment to "a form of hope which at end-of-life is lost" (Sullivan, 2003, p. 394). That is, it is too late to aspire to rectify psychological damage that, as in Diski's case, is long-established and entrenched. However, as Sullivan observes, and as is discussed in Theme iii) above, as long as a trusting interpersonal environment has already been fostered around them, here-and-now work with the despairing and lost can be especially beneficial in the heightened atmosphere of a time of crisis.

Recommendation

Dying individuals still carrying intransigent issues of abandonment and despair may not be helped by a one-to-one therapy, which may take years to yield results. On the other hand, dying is a time of crisis in which people can sometimes become aware of, and work with, normally inaccessible issues. Accordingly, if someone were astute enough to recognise the despair felt by individuals like Diski, there is a class of short-term, specialised therapeutic interventions which might be beneficial to them. Medical psychologists, Gum and Snyder, advocate the use of a therapy intended to generate hope in the dying; the emphasis is on restoring respect for their sense of agency which, for the despairing generally and certainly for Diski, would be a positive move. Rather than being directed towards improving the patient's continued life, Gum and Snyder's program is intended to minister to their most urgent issue, their "dying pathway" (Gum & Snyder, 2002, p. 883).

Theme (viii) Tactics for managing distress about facing death

Survival mechanisms had to be found on receiving a cancer diagnosis, and all participants developed tactics for managing their distress. Gould already had a repertoire of ploys, such as visualising his fears as enemies which could be batted away; this allowed him to change his mood, so that his fear and apprehension were replaced by his usual sense of being in charge of events. Hitchens and Mayne both shut down an early tendency to self-pity, believing that when they most needed to be strong, it could only bring them down. Taylor maintained a feeling of control by keeping a suicide drug to hand, and found distraction and comfort in meetings with a Buddhist nun, whom she found serene and calming. Having few skills of self-care or emotional self-regulation, Diski was reliant on frangible and short-lived mantras, such as reminding herself that she had been "not here" before (Diski, p. 149), or that millions had been through death and dying before her.

Many papers have been written about management of the distress felt by terminal cancer sufferers, and a number of them report how steadying it can be to dying patients to feel in control of their destiny; rather than 'going it alone', they can benefit from constructively sharing activities with their treating professionals. For example, Parkes et al. note that, along with truthful information about their condition, all patients should be given the reliable assurance that they can contact an appropriate doctor "at any time" (Parkes et al., 1996, p.85). As seen in Chapter 6, Part II. *Attitude to medical professionals*, even Diski had found that being free to do this enabled her to contain her anxiety, and to continue with her treatment. A study by Schroepfer, Noh and Kavanaugh (2009) found that patients could adapt more positively to being terminally ill by being shown how they could choose to change their attitudes to it, as Gould had done. In the same vein, as Parkes et al. observe, some patients could even become more optimistic in mood on learning from their doctors that, by the time their condition was terminal, "for them, the worst was over" (Parkes et al., 1996, p. 87).

Recommendation

Although for terminal patients, dying is usually understood to be inevitable, the fear and grief that they feel can be alleviated if medical professionals are supportive enough, and the patients are actively involved in the management of their condition. As Patrick, Engelberg and Curtis note, there is much for patients nearing the end of life to reflect on, and to make decisions about with significant others; for example, they need to decide on what treatments they now wish to give up, or to choose how to die and with whom present – or not present. Above all, they need to be recognised as "a whole person", and "to keep [their] ... dignity and self-respect" (Patrick et al., 2001, p. 721). The over-arching theme of all of these contributions is that, until death comes, the dying still have a life to live, and within the limitations imposed by their illness, it is of the essence to their peace of mind that their condition is not experienced as a premature death-in-life.

Theme (ix) Strategies for maintaining long-term support

As distinct from tactics to manage shorter-term periods of distress, all participants could rely on support from their spouses, families and friends, as well as in Taylor's case, Exit International, and in Mayne's, God, and religious communities, to strengthen their resources over the long haul.

Recommendation

Clearly, for patients lacking family or friends to support them, other means of sustaining themselves need to be found. Though there may be individuals who do not want to tell others about their illness, dying of cancer alone would not be likely to be the preferred choice of most people. Long-term, regularly-meeting groups run by professional leaders of the kind referred to above could offer solitary individuals the companionship and support of a group, and the possibility of friendship with other members, whom they know can really understand what they are going through.

Fourth cluster: Psychological issues and their management

This cluster is made up of three themes.

Theme (x) Radical disbelief versus denial

A concept original to this study, *radical disbelief,* ensues when a terminal condition unexpectedly discovered during a routine examination is diagnosed, but because it fails to connect with the recipient's still symptom-free sense of being-in-life, it does not resonate, and therefore, is not taken on board. Given that the patient's being in a state of radical disbelief is neither a disagreement with the diagnosis, nor a refusal to discuss it, doctors breaking the bad news may not be aware that their patient is in its grip. And yet, now that advanced medical technology can reveal previously unsuspected anomalies, radical disbelief may not be uncommon; indeed, of the full total of six participants in the study, two experienced radical disbelief – Diski, and the author. Moreover, as in Diski's case, a radical disbelief which is not detected by the doctor can hinder a patient's commitment to a treatment regimen; as a result, they might be thought unco-operative, or even be written off when in fact, what they need is for their doctor to be positively concerned about their seeming lack of relatedness to their condition.

As the patient will not dispute the diagnosis in either case, radical disbelief cannot immediately be distinguished from genuine denial. One way of tackling this problem would be to find a way to discard the possibility of the patient being in denial, before testing their commitment to the reality of the diagnosis. Genuine denial cannot be discovered by direct questioning, but it can be detected, for example, in what a patient says when asked about his or her plans after having surgery, and leaving hospital. If in denial, at some point the patient will be likely to express unrealistic ideas like rejoining a football team, or going overseas to a country with primitive medical facilities. Radical disbelief, on the other hand, might be suspected if, like Diski, a patient complains that it is only the treatment that makes them unwell, or seems obsessed with details of their case without seeming able to internalise what they are told. Typically, the specialist would have a sense of not properly connecting with such a patient.

Recommendation

A way needs to be found to link the patient with their illness – as Diski put it: "Everything is presented to me statistically, as probabilities. I can't find the right question to break through that, to talk about the cancer that is me and mine … how it and I are with each other" (Diski, p. 117). What is needed is for the doctor to identify the patient's *own experience* of symptoms like pain, or breathlessness, and to link this with a clear explanation of how this is an effect of their cancer, and then, explain until the patient has understood it, how a proposed treatment can make a difference to their symptoms.

Theme (xi) Problems with prognoses based on statistical probability

Prognoses necessarily based on statistical probabilities as Diski's was, can create serious ambiguities; in comparison with the individualised assessments of the stage of their cancer and its probable future behaviour received by the other four participants, for patients like Diski, the prognosis was disconcertingly vague. With this uncertainty always in the background, it is more difficult for the patient to understand with any confidence how long they have to live, leaving them with a hazy real-time sense of the time available for them to carry out special projects, and say goodbye to significant people. Moreover, their lacking clarity about how long they have to prepare for death could interfere with the developmental process of readying themselves for it. These ambiguities lead in turn to a further problem, the undermining of the patient's sense of agency; such an absence of basic certainties may even leave the patient unsure if the life they are still inhabiting really belongs to them.

Recommendation

Since nothing can be done to rectify the nature of the prognosis, any intervention would need to target its consequences; amongst these, the loss of a sense of agency is a core issue. Indian American surgeon Atul Gawande's approach to patients recognises them as agents from the beginning. His focus is on what those facing mortality want, rather than on how long they have to live, and which treatments will extend it – questions with diminished relevance to people with vague prognoses in any case. Instead, he always asks patients the same five questions, all of which address the patient-as-agent: What do you understand of where you are, and of your illness? What are your fears and worries for the future? What are your goals and priorities? What outcomes are acceptable to you, and what are you willing to sacrifice, or not? and What would a good day look like? (Campbell, 2015, pp. 2–4).

Clarke, Korotchenko and Bundon cite sociologist Victor Marshall's program as supporting agency in a different, but related way. He also advocates asking, rather than telling, dying patients what they may have on their agendas:

i) 'legitimation of biography' – reflecting on one's life history to achieve some kind of coherence, personal meaning and closure
ii) 'legitimation of death' – enabling older adults to view their impending deaths as an appropriate, acceptable and desirable end to their biographies

iii) 'authorship or status control' focuses on the idea that individuals want to be in control of their lives as they end (as cited in Clarke et al., 2012, p. 1412)

Theme (xii) Creative disregard

An important factor in negotiating a period of grave or terminal illness is the ability, while a patient is still well enough, to move away from preoccupation with the illness, and immerse themselves in a cherished activity. It may be travelling the home country as a 'Grey nomad', learning a language or, like the participants in this study, writing a book sharing their experience for the interest and edification of others. A further concept original to this study, *creative disregard* occurs when an individual is able to set aside the anger and distress of contracting a calamitous illness, and find the peace of mind and joy of creativity to invest in life away from painful immediate concerns. Creative disregard does not involve denial; indeed, the approach of death is never far from consciousness, and that it must have its due is never in dispute. The capacity for creative disregard seems to depend on one's having a perspective on life in which the self is no longer at its centre but rather, is part of the world of others, and of the ongoing narrative of the planet; the time is coming to let one's own individual life go. Unlike the other participants, however, Diski could not address the world of others in this way; as she herself observed regarding her work in general, her memoir never moved far away from a stable preoccupation with herself. Accordingly, although infinitely rewarding for those who can embrace it in their final months or years, creative disregard is by no means an automatic rite of passage.

It is not known what proportion of the dying have the capacity for creative disregard; after all, the study participants were accomplished writers. What is known is that, in terms of development of character and personal insights, the dying do regularly break new ground; it is possible, therefore, that they would respond positively to events designed to stimulate creative activity.

Recommendation

Breitbart, Rosenfeld, Gibson, Pessin, Poppito, Nelson ... and Olden trialled a short-term program that they called, "Meaning-centred group psychotherapy", intended to sustain or enhance a sense of meaning, peace and purpose for patients nearing death from advanced cancer (Breitbart et al., 2010, p. 21). Based on Viktor Frankl's philosophical and therapeutic writings, the program utilised didactics, discussion and experiential exercises; each of its eight sessions focused on a different theme, such as what the subjects would consider a good or meaningful death, or how they would place their lives in a personal and historical context. Although the program did not reduce psychological distress as much as the concurrent supportive group psychotherapy program did, its subjects claimed to have an improved sense of spiritual well-being and an enhanced sense of meaning – a finding which, at the two-month follow-up point, had become even more marked. Exercising the capacity for intellectual and creative work, or creative disregard, did not reduce psychological distress in the present investigation either; the two states continued to co-exist. Perhaps, though, the sorrow and anger about one's life coming to an end can have a positive side; rather than being solely symptomatic of distress or disappointment, for some individuals, it may also stimulate a final burst of creativity.

Fifth cluster: Living with cancer

This cluster is made up of three themes.

Theme (xiii) Cancer as a metaphor for death

All participants suffered anxiety and grief about facing death; while Hitchens, Taylor and Diski received terminal diagnoses at the outset, and Gould and Mayne received theirs much later in the piece, the knowledge that they had advanced cancer seemed to stimulate death anxiety equally in them all. In comparison with heart conditions, for example, which can often be treated effectively and its casualties returned to reasonable health and normal function sometimes for many years, cancer is known for its recurrence; breaks from it are usually called 'remissions', not cures. Cancer may not be regarded as the inevitable killer that it once was, but for most people, it is still a frightening messenger, either of death, or at the very least, of the need to have harsh treatment with no guarantee of a cure. Nonetheless, leaving people diagnosed with cancer either in ignorance or falsely reassured, is not acceptable; further symptoms will continue to occur, perhaps leaving the patient aware that the truth has been withheld, and fearful that it must be thought to be too terrible to tell them.

Recommendation

If they ask him, Matthew O'Reilly, crisis ambulance paramedic, always tells gravely-ill people that they are dying. In his experience, they make full use of the short time they have left; they usually accept the news quietly, often seek forgiveness for wrongdoings, wish to be remembered to loved ones, and try to reflect on the meaning of their lives (O'Reilly, 2014, September 25, YouTube broadcast). Parkes et al. believe that, whether the patient asks for the diagnosis or not, to leave them in ignorance robs them of knowing that their time is limited, and that they need to prepare themselves for death. Where possible, having chosen the best time and place to do it, the doctor should tell patients as much as they can take in, and especially, "listen for unasked questions" (Parkes et al., 1996, p. 80).

Theme (xiv) Dying in one's sixties should not happen

Hitchens, Gould and Taylor all found themselves facing death from cancer when they were in their early sixties; as opposed to older participants, Diski (67) and Mayne (76), who felt no responsibility for developing cancer, these three participants all blamed themselves for having done so. Certainly, dying in one's early sixties is today often considered untimely, and those who do, examples of deaths which were premature or perhaps, should not have happened at all. Amongst the hypotheses circulating in the public health domain at present, notions that there must have been a failure of 'right living' involved are not hard to find. Drinking more than a specified amount of alcohol, smoking, eating processed foods or too much salt, neglect of cholesterol levels, and avoiding exercise all rank as delinquent practices, from which we can only expect to sicken, and in all likelihood, eventually die. Nowadays, insurance companies often exact higher premiums from such 'guilty parties' for income protection and life insurance, or even refuse to insure them at all. An example of the creation of a class of such 'guilty parties' for public consumption was demonstrated in Work Cover advertisements on television a few years ago, in which the father of three young children is pictured coughing up blood from his putative cigarette smoking-caused lung cancer. Most striking of all is how haunted by guilt he looks; the advertisement implies that, by selfishly indulging in smoking, he is dying an avoidable death and therefore, he is to blame for abandoning his family to an uncertain and fatherless future.

Recommendation

It is concerning that public health advice which was initially planned as a supportive guide to wellness, can at times be unhelpfully skewed. The kind of publicity that over-simplifies the way illnesses like lung cancer develop, and sends a message blaming people for getting sick, should be avoided. Given that denial and the consequent failure to seek help flourish on feelings of guilt, shame and resentment, such presentations of public health messages should be replaced by a non-judgmental, factual and informative approach.

Theme (xv) Effectiveness of programs for self-monitoring of cancer symptoms

All participants had warnings of the presence in their bodies of serious cancer symptoms. Some, like Mayne and Taylor, had well-developed cancers, which for too long they had neglected to have checked out. Others, like Gould, Hitchens and Diski, had warnings from ongoing health problems that all was far from well; Diski's pulmonary fibrosis was already being monitored. As educated, well-off people, the participants would have been aware of public health advice about self-monitoring and reporting of cancer symptoms, but none had done so. Indeed, in general, while there are people who say that checking for cancer symptoms led them to seek screening, apparently, many do not do so. In 2020 to 2021, for example, the participation rates for females in breast cancer screening in the targeted age group of fifty to seventy-four, was only 48% (*National Cancer Control Indicators*, 2020–2021, July 15, 2022. Retrieved from ncci.canceraustralia.gov.au/screening/breast-screening-rates/breast-screening-rates).

It might be thought that we need more information or perhaps, more pressure from our doctors to invest in self-monitoring of symptoms, but perhaps it is simply too much to ask. In our society, cancer is often understood to be a metaphor for a harrowing death; committing ourselves to the self-surveillance required by cancer checks faces us with a cruel dilemma. We might be lucky this time and find nothing, but next time, or the next, we might not be so lucky; a comparison with placing ourselves beneath the sword of Damocles does not seem completely out of place.

Recommendation

Given that the self-monitoring procedure is often not easy to carry out, and that we are fearful of finding something suspect – or of not knowing whether it is or not – self-monitoring is also likely to be unreliable; it may well be preferable for us to be checked out by someone who has medical expertise. Accordingly, it is suggested that health programs providing medical check-ups for possible cancer symptoms be widened to include more types of cancer, and that the public be facilitated in using them; self-monitoring could be explicitly allocated a secondary role, and seeking check-ups by health professionals encouraged as preferable.

Equally importantly, to encourage people to regulate self-damaging activities and to volunteer to be checked, messages of hope are needed. For example, when urged to quit smoking, many people may feel guiltily that it is already too late, or that reversing the damage will be too slow for them to reap much benefit. Accordingly, they may be reassured that quitting is worthwhile if they are informed that human lungs begin to regenerate immediately after quitting; ten years later, the damage to all organs will be significantly reduced, and fifteen years later, almost completely removed (*Medical News Today Newsletter*, 2018, November 9. Retrieved from healthline.com/health/what-happens-when-you-quit-smoking).

Part II. Themes relating to study question 2. If our most basic instinct is to survive, how can we become ready to relinquish life and accept death?

Sixth cluster: Attitudes to dying

This is a single-theme cluster.

Theme (xvi) Imagining dying

All participants tried to imagine what dying would be like, and apart from Hitchens, expressed a probably common enough fear of dying; it would mean encountering the unknown and unknowable. Eventually, Mayne found security in his relationship with God, Taylor eased herself into a gentle feeling of returning in her mother's care to inchoate oblivion; Gould stared his fear down, and fearing a death while delusional, Hitchens vowed to stay with the facts of his now arduous reality. All four participants who appeared to have followed their own inner direction in letting their fears go, became ready to prepare for dying. On the other hand, having always maintained control through knowing things and thus, having avoided depending on trust, Diski could not accept that she need not, and indeed, could not know in advance how to die. Unlike the other four participants, she appeared to have no access to an inner process that she knew she could trust to direct her.

Individuals like Diski seem to have experienced a failure of normal maturation which, albeit after a struggle, allows us to realise that dying is the natural end to our lives. Moreover, resources to help individuals who are unprepared for death may not be readily available. Discussing the failure of medical systems to address the chronically and terminally ill about dying, Price and Cheek quote Kellehear (2007), as observing: "Dying cannot be made good or managed if there is no recognition of dying" (as cited in Price & Cheek, 2007, p. 403). That is, if an individual continues to receive only the same unhelpful advice about coping with their illness and their dying is never mentioned, they may actually be handicapped in their attempts to prepare for it.

Recommendation

Essentially, what patients unprepared for dying need is not knowledge, but to feel safe. As well as needing to be talked to supportively and often about dying, their sometime regression to feeling like a frightened child requires attention. Kuhl points out that the dying in general crave physical contact, both for comfort, and to counteract a feeling of being untouchable: "Touch is supportive of self-esteem and bodily connectedness" (Kuhl, 2003, p. 99). Accordingly, as long as they are able to sit with them, talk to them and if it is wanted, hold their hands, empathic medical professionals like Diski's trusted Nurse L. might be able to make frightened patients like Diski feel a little safer as they die.

Seventh cluster: Attitudes facing imminent death

This cluster has three themes.

Theme (xvii) Attitudes facing impending death

As death approached, the five participants each faced it in their own way. Mayne was steadfast and ready to die, and though anguished about the forthcoming parting from his wife, he felt close to God. In a state of quasi-mystical ecstasy, Gould was feeling strong, and ready to die. Taylor was composed, but she missed that special person to be with her at her death – her mother perhaps; however, gently drifting away, she was ready to return to being part of the universe. Hitchens was no longer intimidated by dying, but now increasingly aware of his vulnerabilities, he was determined not to die giving in to them. Dying had changed all the participants – for four of them, in the direction of rendering them more the person they already were, and had the potential to become. Diski alone remained unready and terrified.

As individuals, the participants all reacted differently to dying but at the same time, overall, very much as human beings have faced death from time immemorial.

Recommendation

A recommendation is needed for only one participant, Diski; her needs facing imminent death have been discussed in the section immediately above: *Imagining dying*.

Theme (xviii) Sustaining the self as death approaches

As they had done at diagnosis, the participants met dying in their characteristic ways. When her hospice did not guarantee her a place when her time to die came, Diski closed down. Afraid that sympathy from others and his own sorrow would threaten his self-control, Hitchens also withdrew. On the other hand, as they had done throughout, Mayne, Gould and Taylor remained engaged with others to the end.

It is possible that those who need to withdraw might unintentionally cause distress to their loved ones. When they recall that the dying person is behaving exactly as they always have in a crisis, however, survivors may find some solace at the seeming rejection. However, the loss of the opportunity to be intimately with the dying other as they would have wished, is likely to be harder to accept.

Recommendation

To address this concern, survivors might first be encouraged to recall ways in which the other's withdrawals were dealt with in the past; then, those which can be adapted to offer comfort both to the loved one and to themselves, can become a here-and-now resource. Stanley and Wise (2011, see Chapter 2, Part III: *Turning a blind eye to death: Sequestering the dying*) discuss the conversion of long-established domestic practices into new and transformative responses to the dying of a family member. Such an adaptation in this case might include remaining quietly present, while playing music the dying person had in life found comforting at times of stress.

Theme (xix) Life-prolonging treatment versus quality time

For cancer sufferers, a decision to accept medical treatments to prolong life often results in the detriment of its quality. Nonetheless, Hitchens and Gould accepted all treatments that were offered; Hitchens resisted losing even one moment of life, while Gould was writing a book on politics that he was determined to finish. Having completed it, however, and convinced that the right time for him to die had come, he wanted no more treatment for the cancer, although he did accept antibiotics for the infection which finally took his life. Once in receipt of a terminal diagnosis and with three months to live, Mayne rejected further chemotherapy in favour of quality of life; Diski considered terminating chemotherapy to avoid a further deterioration in her quality of life. Taylor refused life-prolonging treatment at the end in favour of quality of death. In all, three participants were concerned about the ill-effects of treatment with two, possibly three, deciding more life was not worth the loss of its quality; another participant refused further treatment because he felt that it was the right time to die, and finally, the last participant, who above all valued being alive, accepted all the treatments he was given to the end.

The assumption that all dying people will want to extend life as far as possible does not appear to reflect reality, and it would not be a reliable basis on which to work out the funding of treatment programs. A more nuanced collection of data would be required to obtain accurate, and possibly more modest figures.

Amongst the public health programs that these findings might illuminate, Advance Care Planning stands out. Given the variety of attitudes to medical intervention even in this study's sample of five, tickbox or other forms of one-size-fits-all Advance Care Planning would appear less than fit for purpose.

Recommendation

Flexible, ongoing discussion with GPs, or even as late as the final stage of life, with ICU staff will be needed if people are to plan the kind of death they would most hope to have. Taylor's experience shows that all ambiguities inevitably present in Advance Care Planning formats need to be worked through by people making Plans. With so many factors in play, it can be difficult to identify preferences in the manner of one's dying, even in the grip of a terminal disease; making Advance Care Plans some time before a final illness is even known to be in the offing, however, might be no better than guesswork or wishful thinking.

Eighth cluster: Rites of passage in accepting death

This cluster has five themes.

Theme (xx) Prelude: Towards acceptance of death

Four participants were able to accept dying; only Diski could not. According to Gould: "I believe that only when you accept death can you free yourself from it. Acceptance is the key" (Gould, p. 118); to Mayne: "We each choose to die in our own way but if we can see it as a gift, it will be, insofar as we can let go of what we have been given with open hands" (Mayne, pp. 250–251); from Hitchens, now that he is dying, a declaration that he must above all, avoid succumbing to fantasy and wishful thinking, and from Taylor, now that she has accepted that dying is an inescapable part of life, an assurance that she finds that good things can come of it. In Diski's case, an internal directive particular to her had overwritten the path to acceptance; it seems to have been something like: "Trust no one, always call the shots yourself".

Accepting death seems to involve accessing an innate inscription that dying is as natural as being born. Rather than being contacted by reasoning, or even by spiritual understanding, acceptance seems to be a state of being, an awareness which is typically activated in mature human beings when they experience the approach of death. To access the inscription that dying is natural and requires no particular expertise, time is needed, but it can take place as well over a long time of dying, like Taylor's, or over a very short one, as ambulance veteran Matthew O'Reilly revealed in Living with cancer, *Theme xiii* above. As is discussed in the remainder of this cluster, however, access to death acceptance may become blocked if certain preparatory work cannot be done.

No recommendations are made at this preliminary stage.

Theme (xxi) Tangible items: Putting one's affairs in order

There were no tasks considered essential by all participants, though Wills, financial and business matters, funerals and bodily disposal were attended to by all three men and by Taylor. Gould and Mayne wrote letters of farewell to their families at the time of their first surgery, as did Taylor, though given that her letter explained her suicidal intent if the surgery ended badly, she did not deliver it. Diski did not report making any preparations; in satirical vein, she drew up a parody of the usual funeral format. However, like Taylor, she did make an Advance Care Plan to try to ensure as comfortable a death as possible. For Gould, the most significant item to finalise was finding the right grave plot in a well-known cemetery, chosen to accommodate the visitors he expected would meet there.

Recommendation

As can be seen from the assortment of customary and idiosyncratic activities that mattered to the participants, adequate time and someone trusted and willing to assist with their plans without judgment, will always be needed by the dying. Like Diski, some individuals may need someone else to take care of their affairs.

Theme (xxii) Intangible items 1. Resolution of conflicts

All five participants had unfinished business involving conflict with others, or within themselves; in all cases, there was a compelling need to resolve it.

For Mayne, Taylor and Diski, the conflict was intrapersonal, with an internal parent or their equivalent; in each case, it showed itself through an issue which, while it did not immediately advertise what the core problem was, caught and held the participants' attention.

For Diski, the alert came in her obsessive examinations and re-examinations of her failed relationship with Peter and Doris Lessing. She did not realise that she was trapped in an endless re-enactment of her relationship with her abusive parents, and that this was why she was so caught up in a state of distrust and rage. She could neither forgive them or herself, nor cut them loose.

For Mayne, the alert came from his relationship to icons of Jesus. He had always been a devotee of tenderly-smiling icons – arguably, the obverse of his image of his suicide father – but through finding himself irresistibly drawn to an icon of the suffering and at times, stern, but always faithful, Gethsemane Jesus, Mayne began to realise that at last, he could think of his father with forbearance, and without judgment. Once aware of this, he underwent a painful confrontation with himself, emerging as an advocate of standing up to, but not condemning, those we feel have wronged us. Having understood this, he became a protective and resolute father to himself and his family; while ready to listen to medical authorities, he made his own decisions.

For Taylor, the alert came from her indecision about whether or not to take her suicide drug. She was afraid of suffering a terrible death over which she had no control, and although the drug represented her insurance against such a catastrophe, she continued to hesitate over taking it. Finally, she became aware that what she was really afraid of was having so damaged the internal memory of her mother, that she could not hope to call on her in her hour of need, and as a consequence, would feel abandoned to die alone and in anguish. In fact, she seems to have experienced a gentle, dreamy drift towards death, with her caring husband in attendance; her final words show that the sense of her mother's loving presence did return to her.

For Gould and Hitchens, the conflict was interpersonal, with other people. For Gould, the alert came when his wife confronted him with his arrogant dismissal of her homemaking achievements, and with having continually moved the family on to suit his work arrangements. Gould recognised that this was true, and was empathically and profoundly sorry. His wife forgave him, and they remained close until his death.

For Hitchens, the alert came when he came under attack by Christian believers, who had heard about his cancer, rejoiced in it and had begun to circulate rumours that he had recanted his antitheism on his deathbed. He devoted the first chapter of his memoir to denouncing their beliefs, and reiterating his rejection of their claim that he had recanted his antitheism.

It is widely understood that the dying may need to attend to unfinished business – often involving the issue of forgiving, or not forgiving, the self and others – and that they seek to right wrongs before they die. What may be less well-known is that, when apparently unrelated events or objects like choice of icons, or euthanasia drugs kept 'just in case', repeatedly demand the attention of a dying person, they are likely to be a clue to some fundamental issue below the surface of consciousness that needs attention. Resolution of conflicts like this may be essential to the process of death acceptance.

Recommendation

In the present study, four out of five participants resolved the conflicted issue themselves, which suggests that in the ordinary way, the intensity of the experience of dying may enable many individuals to work out even deeply repressed issues on their own, or with the help of family and friends. For those who cannot do so, however, the situation may become grave; in that case, specialist help might be sought, and in the high-pressure atmosphere of dying, it may be uniquely effective.

Theme (xxiii) Intangible items 2. Deathbed confessions

Only three participants recorded a final confidence near the end of their memoirs – Diski, Gould and Taylor. All three outlined what they saw as a dark area in their psyche – Diski to portray her core self as without gratitude to, or love for anyone; Gould to acknowledge that he might be thought to be – and perhaps was – arrogant and opinionated, especially in his critique of his first surgery, and Taylor, after abandoning her mother in an institution, to reveal how she yearned to know that she was not in her turn abandoned.

Making a confession traditionally implies a quest for absolution, and in a sense, that is occurring here; the listener is not God's representative, but an authority figure that each confessing party has created. Gould's internal confessor agrees with him that he is arrogant, but does so without judgment; Gould has been advised that other specialists support his latest campaign, which is to tell the truth about his famous but insufficiently competent doctor: "I would do it all again", he declares (Gould, p. 132). Taylor's yearning cry for her mother conveys her regret, but at the same time, the hope of being heard. As seen in the next section, her final words show that she believed that she was heard. By contrast with the previous two participants, when she presents herself convincingly enough as the horrible child nobody wants, Diski imagines her internal confessor as worse than unforgiving; hers appears to be unresponsive and menacing. Thus, where Taylor and Gould can feel accepted and move forward towards acceptance, Diski cannot.

Recommendation

For individuals like Diski, because the inner other is unforgiving or threatening, their inner world lacks humanity and tenderness. It is important not to remonstrate with any such individual, or to suggest that a caring presence must surely be there somewhere; they would probably turn away in scorn, but underlying that, in despair. While quietly listening to them is of the first importance if they are to feel accepted as they are, entering into their tragic world is generally to be avoided. In the dynamic time of dying, a direct, empathic and kind approach to them in what they are facing in the here and now may be the best way to provide them with the comfort and support they need, but may not be able to ask for.

Theme (xxiv) Acceptance, or redemption

Access to the inscription for acceptance of dying seems to be governed by two main factors. Firstly, the access has to be clear; to become available to the individual, it cannot be overwritten by something more compelling, perhaps originally installed to protect someone's survival and by now, an unconscious directive; an example of this would be: "No one can be trusted". Secondly, the resolution of crucial conflicts is essential to the quietness of mind necessary to end the restless searching for vindication, and accept letting go. Confession is not a necessary part of reaching acceptance in itself, but it can provide clues as to whether or not the way to acceptance is clear. In the event that, for reasons of personal history, the access is blocked, it is suggested that an alternative path to an unpersecuted death may be found if like Diski, in her unsparing love for her grandchildren, the individual undergoes a redemptive experience.

Recommendation

No matter how eccentric or even bizarre it may seem, if a redemptive process is spontaneously occurring, it is not necessary to intervene. As has been suggested, when her psychic pain became intolerable, Diski's love for her grandchildren may have brought about such a redemptive experience, in the form of a self-protective breakdown. In such a case, caution should be exercised about pressing for the individual to return to reality; if a much-needed refuge has been provided by the breakdown, that would need to be respected.

Ninth cluster: Spirituality

This cluster has two themes.

Theme (xxv) Experiences of a spiritual dimension

As a loyal and sincere Anglican, Mayne had been spiritually active and aware throughout his life. As he neared death, his faith became stronger, and his sense of God's concern profound. Also a long-term Anglican, Gould was increasingly disappointed in his church's response to him when he found himself *in extremis*; he became sceptical of its spiritual understanding and instead, once in the Death Zone, he was guided by his own mystical experience. Taylor remained an atheist until she died, but she had an inchoate sense of the importance of the sacred; drawn to the serenity of a Buddhist nun she had met, she decided to ask the nun to say some prayers for the dead at her funeral. Neither Diski, an atheist, nor Hitchens, an antitheist, had any time for religious or spiritual thinking or cosmology. In fact, none of the three atheist participants expressed concern about their irreligious views, or sought to espouse a more reverent attitude because they were dying.

Recommendation

People who are not conventionally religious may nonetheless wish to observe some element of the sacred in their passing.

Theme (xxvi) Christians compared with atheists facing death

Facing imminent death, Christians Mayne and Gould saw nothing in themselves that should be radically overhauled in order to meet God in the afterlife; they looked forward to it with humility but also, with joyous anticipation. On the other hand, facing death, atheist Diski felt that, despite all of her literary achievements, her life had been of no consequence and might just as well never have happened. And while atheist Taylor regarded her thriving sons and her successful books as deeply satisfying contributions to this world, she talked about her ashes being "tossed out" by her husband as if, now no longer being useful, she had become nothing but a disposable remnant (Taylor, p. 105). Believing self-pity and responding to empathic concern to be mere sentimentality, antitheist Hitchens vowed, as he prepared to meet his end, neither to express vulnerability himself, nor to respond emotionally to any demonstrations of compassion and sympathy by anyone else.

It is striking that, with death now imminent, those who attributed perfection to an external being saw no need for self-improvement before their first encounter with the deity, while those who denied the existence of any such being, judged themselves more negatively; perhaps the reverse arrangement might have been a more logical expectation? It might be argued that Diski's history, Hitchens' tough stance to meet death, and Taylor's references to being "tossed out", can all be fully accounted for in terms of what is known about each of them as persons, and there can be no doubt that personal factors shaped the severity of their attitudes towards themselves. Nonetheless, although this is a small sample, it may suggest that, in this secular age, perhaps a price is being paid by the dying for their loss of external objects of worship. Not only do the unbelieving have to face the lack of an afterlife and of a compassionate deity, but also, while their *achievements* in life may remain, at life's end *they themselves* seem to have little value – neither intrinsic, nor even accrued. Elias (1985) has argued that, taken out of the context of meaningful attachments, death in modernity has become meaningless, no matter how fulfilling the life may have been. But the picture for these unbelievers seems even more negative than that; these three participants appeared to see themselves as some kind of leftovers, awaiting disposal with whatever stoicism they could muster.

A study by Neimeyer, Wittkowski and Moser of individuals who had endorsed death-acceptance, found that they were more able to see meaning in death when they could put it into "an over-arching concept of some kind" (Neimeyer et al., 2004, p. 334). Moreover, being able to invest in such a meaningful framework also seemed to help them to experience less fear about personal death.

Recommendation

While Neimeyer et al.'s perhaps unsurprising conclusion is relevant to the experience of dying believers, it does not explain the tentative findings of the present study that atheistic individuals show some negativity towards their personal value when dying. Although such small numbers are involved, the result does show a clear and consistent demarcation between the two groups; accordingly, a further in-depth investigation of this result could be rewarding.

Tenth cluster: What is meaningful to the dying participants

This cluster has two themes.

Theme (xxvii) Love

Apart from Diski's antagonism towards Doris Lessing and Hitchens' towards his Christian adversaries, every participant wrote about love and very little about animosity. Gould believed that his last months on earth were to be spent giving as much love as he could to his family and beyond, to all creation; Hitchens adored his work and conversation with his friends; Mayne loved his family and friends, and believed that he and his God loved each other unconditionally; Taylor loved her husband and sons and especially, her mother; Diski did not believe herself capable of love, but she wept over the impending loss of her grandchildren.

No recommendation is required by this finding.

Theme (xxviii) Creativity, with a touch of immortality

Every participant also wrote about the importance to them of their creativity, as represented in their writings. Further, in the sense of leaving something of themselves for generations still to come, Gould, Mayne and Taylor hoped for the touch of the immortality that is conferred by one's work being recognised and remembered. Neither Hitchens nor Diski expressed any such expectation; Hitchens merely hoped that his words would protect people from succumbing to the self-righteously pious at least in the immediate future, and

Diski, that her grandchildren would remember her from photographs and stories. However, the participants were united on one point; for those who can do so, to support ongoing living and especially, to avoid becoming lost in the ravages of the illness and its treatment, investing in some kind of creative activity is essential. This finding suggests that, even if they were not artists or writers, other chronic or terminally-ill patients could be encouraged to use their imaginations to open up their horizons, and in so doing, help to prevent themselves from being trapped in their disease.

Recommendation

A model for how such encouragement might be provided, UK oncology nurse, Ellen Carr, devised a program intended to restore hope, and to help patients to think beyond the hospital ward. Using documentaries and films, she found that stories of salvation such as *The Shawshank redemption,* and televised talks from inspirational people like Olivia Newton-John and Betty Ford, greatly lifted patients' spirits. Both of these women then had cancer diagnosed for the second time, but "were not just giving up and starting to die"; their "go ahead and live" messages were especially powerful and appreciated (Carr, 2008, p. 50). Arguably, Carr's program stimulated in her patients the beginnings of a capacity for *creative disregard.*

Eleventh cluster: Three themes exemplifying gender differences

This cluster has four themes. The first three themes exemplify particular gender differences among the participants, and the fourth provides an overall summarising statement. The recommendation is entered after the fourth theme.

Theme (xxix) Why the participant wrote the memoir

Some objectives in writing the memoir were shared, but all participants had one in particular that was theirs alone. Initially, Diski decided that she had to write a column in the *London review of books* about having cancer; ultimately, however, what she most appreciated was the opportunity for thinking and analysing life events and relationships that the writing had given her.

Taylor, like Diski, wanted to use writing the memoir for herself; her aim was to provide an outline of her death, so that she and others could see it clearly. At the same time, she found that being absorbed in analysing life events and telling the reader something meaningful, prevented her mind and attention from locking on to her body's descent into catastrophe.

First published in *The Times*, Gould originally wrote his memoir to show people that it is possible to suffer cancer, and emerge stronger. Once given a terminal diagnosis, his objective became to enable them to overcome the fear of death. He did not identify a direct therapeutic value for himself in writing the memoir, but his reflections about the illness and his responses to it suggest that he did find writing his memoir a positive experience.

Hitchens loved to write articles, usually with polemical intent. In particular, he wanted the first chapter of his memoir to stand in permanent rebuttal of Christian dogma and of the rumour his opponents had started that, once terminally-ill, he had turned for succour to Christianity. He also believed that in general, hospital procedures could be poorly administered and that therefore, they needed to be monitored.

Mayne's memoir was in part, a cancer journal, and in part, a set of essays on spiritual matters. It had two functions: firstly, it was to be a record of how his beliefs stood the test of his having cancer, and secondly, in sharing his experience honestly with others, it was intended to offer them comfort, companionship, and validation of their feelings.

For the three male participants, the memoir's main purpose was as a kind of mission statement; they all intended to inform and in doing so, to educate and benefit their readers. Mayne also wanted to monitor how his beliefs stood up to his having cancer. By contrast, for the two women, the memoirs were focused on their introspections about personal matters, and analysing their relationships.

Theme (xxx) How the participants relate to medical professionals

Hitchens, Gould and Mayne were mainly positive about their medical professionals, while Diski and Taylor were mainly negative about them. Hitchens idealised his doctors, regarding them as exceptional and altruistic physicians; he was willing to talk only to them about his illness. Gould described how his first experience of surgery had turned out badly, but reported warmly on his second oncologist as: "[ready to] ... fight with me every inch of the way" (Gould, p. 52). Despite having some brutal and at times, questionable treatment, Mayne trusted his doctors uncritically for quite some time though eventually, he realised that he had to be more selective about both doctors and treatments.

On the other hand, both Taylor and Diski were generally dissatisfied with the medical professionals they encountered, though having found nurses kind, Diski reserved her criticisms for her doctors and the radiographers. While she had no complaints about the treatment she had received from her doctors, Taylor was unpleasantly surprised that none of them spoke to her about her approaching death, or showed any other awareness of her as a person. Diski's complaints were similar. She felt that apart from the nurses, nobody showed any concern or respect for her as an individual; she wondered if they cared more about the technicalities of their machines than about her personal welfare.

The male participants were not concerned with the way doctors related to them as persons; they were satisfied with having their medical care delivered objectively and effectively. By contrast, the women wanted to be approached personally and empathically. In our society, men traditionally distance themselves emotionally from suffering – including their own – while women are more likely to seek, and when needed, to provide, personal support and sympathy when times are troubled.

Having said that, it is interesting to note that, when talking about their doctors, the men speak in an optimistic but surprisingly naïve way, while the women sound disappointed and derisive. Even the normally iconoclastic Hitchens gave his doctors full marks, and both Mayne and Gould accepted ill-advised and inadequate treatment from doctors for some time before deciding that they must be more critical and selective. By contrast, the women were far from naïve about their medical professionals and indeed, were inclined to be downright scathing. For example, Taylor described the death counsellor she saw as radically inadequate for the job: she had left the psychologist's office after the consultation full of scorn, declaring that although the woman was obviously a well-educated whizz kid, all she had to offer were techniques of chilling out that anyone could get from Dr Google. Equally disparagingly, Diski declares: "I don't trust anyone .... What could anyone give me that could definitively improve my health? .... when most of the unwellnesss came from the treatment?" (Diski, p. 207).

Theme (xxxi) Last words of each participant

Diski's final words show that she has become incoherent, but prior to this, she had been writing about her mother's madness and her aggression towards Diski when she reached puberty.

Typically optimistic, Gould wrote: "I am approaching the door marked Death. What lies beyond may be the worst of things. But I believe that it will be the best of things" (Gould, p. 143).

Written the night he died, Hitchens quoted Alan Lightman in praise of mortality: without it, "*No one ever comes into his own* ... Such is the cost of immortality. No person is whole. No person is free" (as cited in Hitchens, pp. 92–93).

Mayne referred to nature, identifying it as the God-given eternal cycle of birth and death: "Each [annual cycle] ... summons us to a sense of wonder at nature's *cantus firmus*. A melody that is both hopeful and enduring" (Mayne, p. 251).

In her final screenplay, Taylor depicted herself reunited with her mother forever: "Movie footage of a girl ... in dappled sunshine ... arm-in-arm with her mother ... crossing the tarmac at an airport .... The jet takes off .... Fade to black" (Taylor, p. 147).

Now ready for death, the men's thoughts turned outwards; they took the form of an optimistic slogan, a universal principle like the law of nature, or a philosophical take on mortality. All three wanted to send a final message to the world. By contrast, the women inclined towards turning inwards, seeking out the mother; doing so left Taylor bathed in happiness, but precipitated Diski into incoherence.

Theme (xxxii) Discussion of gender differences

This investigation is too small to support significant generalisations about gender or any other wide-ranging dispositions in the way people prepare for death. However, across the three sets of findings outlined above, there is a consistency in the direction of their attention by the men as compared with the women; this adds some weight to the finding. From these data, it is evident that the women were drawn inwards, to analysing their feelings and relationships with significant others, especially their mothers or mother-substitutes, while by contrast, the men turned their attention outward, offering principles and guidelines for good living and constructive thinking. The women wanted to understand what motivated both them and others to do what they do, to know what made them tick; they also offered their own ideas about how the work of medical professionals would be improved if they took a personal interest in their patients. By contrast, the men were satisfied with the way the medical services were ordered, content that the doctors were in charge, and satisfied that the object of consultations was the delivery of information and guidance about treatment.

It is possible that the fact that two of the men were titled, and the other was a well-known writer, elicited some special attention and respect from staff. Certainly, the men did not complain that they were treated by their doctors without respect or concern; and yet, even though Diski was also a renowned writer, the women felt belittled. Accordingly, the most potent factor involved in the different attitudes of the men and the women to medical professionals seems to have been gender.

Nevertheless, although it seems quite possible that, like Diski and Taylor, women in general find medical institutions inhospitable, it seems unlikely that anything would readily change in contemporary hospital protocols. Now that the system is a well-established part of our society's structure, many other things would have to happen in the broader fabric of society before such a systemic change in medical circles could take place; arguably, a recommendation pointing to the need for that kind of change would be futile at this stage. If this is right, the seeming naivete of the men about their doctors might be reinterpreted as in part, their unquestioning validation of the hierarchical and rules-based nature of medical organisations, with consultants and administrators – often men – at the top, and the other professionals – where more women work as nurses and allied professionals – assigned to gradually descending other ranks. Accordingly, delivery of health services is likely to remain objective, with little or no place for developing a more personal aspect to professional relationships. For many, even women, this way of organising a medical facility would be familiar, and by and large, at least tolerated.

At the end of life, Taylor and Diski were both preoccupied with their mothers, the former because she missed her loving mother and the latter, because she missed loving mothering itself. While neither was child-like enough to expect to find mother-substitutes in the healthcare system, what they missed from the staff was kindness – a little warmth, and some kindly concern about their condition, and impending death. In its early stages, Diski's treatment and relationship with the hospital had effectively been saved by her experience with kind nurses, especially Nurse L. in the chemotherapy unit. Unfortunately, however, she was then sent on to a series of impersonal and cold treatment environments; partly because of this, and seemingly to the concern of no one, she eventually stopped complying with treatment, and died in a parlous condition two months before the minimum time she had been given to live.

In their book, *Intelligent kindness*, psychiatric specialists Ballatt and Campling (2011) have drawn attention to the gradual disappearance of kindness from NHS establishments, claiming that the inappropriate and increasing use of business models in the delivery of medical care: "works against the idea of an integrated service that prioritises the needs of vulnerable patients", and has put in place: "[a] ... process of industrialising healthcare, in which the skilled attention of its workers being delivered to people who need it is turned into the mechanical delivery of processes and systems" (Ballatt & Campling, 2011, p. 142). Further, they argue that, resentful of the way in which they themselves are treated in a service that emphasises efficient and impersonal practices and at the same time, makes them compete for scarce funding resources, there is a danger of devalued staff falling into perverse practices such as patient neglect, when their professional training would have mandated care and attention.

Recommendation

There can be no immediate alteration to the model used by our society's healthcare systems. Accordingly, within the present system, the recommendation is to maintain and support the value placed upon kindness and empathy in nursing and other caring services, and to promote their availability for all patients who are identified as vulnerable. Both quantity and quality of life are at stake for those who like Diski, are gravely ill, and can be seen to be unable to sustain the harsher elements of treatment without better institutional support.

Part III. *Ars moriendi*: The art of dying well

Human dying resists being defined or treated as a medical management problem rather than as first and foremost, a time for being with loved ones, and for grasping the essence of our lives as we face death, and die. Perhaps there is no such thing as a 'good death' – or at least, not one that can be planned ahead of starting the final journey – but when death takes place in a way which is on our own terms, and captures the unique quality of our lives, dying can be a profoundly sad, and yet a fulfilling and redemptive event for all concerned.

If there is an opportunity for a creative act to accompany it, with every death, an *ars moriendi* can emerge by its own volition. Not limited to celebrations of the passing of the elderly on this occasion, an account of five such events follows.

Dying at home

Mum's goodbye party

Terminally ill with cancer, Mum surprised the family by saying that she wanted a party to say goodbye. Mum had always loved parties, but the family were concerned about whether she would be well enough to cope with one now. Nevertheless, a party was announced; it was to be at 3 PM in the afternoon, so that Mum would be well medicated with what the family called her 'happy pills'- her morphine – but not yet too sleepy to enjoy it.

To Mum, a party involved the guitar and some friends, all singing with her – she knew the words of all of the songs, and she could be relied on to keep the singing going at any party. At this, her final party, she did actually manage to sing along with some of the songs. At other times, her friends would sit with her and hold her arms so that they would wave in time with the music. Alongside the music-making, Mum's friends had the opportunity to be with each other within the framework of Mum's dying experience, and to grieve and mourn together for her, their dear friend, who was soon to leave them forever (Bourgeois & Johnson, 2004, pp. 100–101).

Mum's funerary blanket

On discharge home from hospital with only weeks to live, Mum bought some white wool and gold thread to make a blanket to cover her body while she lay in an open casket at home; she loved doing craft, and crocheted beautifully. For Mum and her family, crocheting a funerary blanket was also crucial to their cultural practices; making the blanket together would involve all of the family and friends who called in to visit Mum, and to accompany her on her last journey. Many of the visitors sat round her bed and crocheted some squares for the blanket; she showed them what ritual required them to do to make the perfect blanket until she was too ill to work on it herself, though she could still oversee and help her assistants. As they worked, they sometimes sang, and at other times, they wept and grieved. Once Mum grew sicker and needed more care, the work became sporadic, and everyone became anxious that the blanket would not be finished in time for Mum to see it. Coming to the rescue, a cousin laboured over the blanket for days in order to finish it in time.

Once finished, the blanket was truly beautiful – a gold-tasselled, white woollen sixty squares – large enough to cover Mum perfectly, and complete with a comfortable pillow, it was described as "perfect for a queen". Finished just a few days before she died, it gave Mum great happiness: "Oh", she exclaimed, "It's beautiful!" It was laid out on a table ready for use, labelled: 'No food or drink, Mum's blanket', and covered with a sheet to keep it clean and safe.

Working together, this network of family and friends had created an atmosphere of safety for its members to begin to grieve, and the completion of the blanket was understood by the family to be a death ritual with a spiritual, as well as a cultural value and importance. Although it was a time of mourning, working together to ensure that Mum's dignity and privacy in death would be respected gave her loved ones deep satisfaction, and a sense of purpose (Bourgeois & Johnson, 2004, p. 102).

Dying in a hospice

Hospice visitor as catalyst

Having been shocked by how blank and bleak funerals were, photographer Tom Murray decided that he had to communicate with people who were dying, to find and draw out the depth of meaning and feeling – the quality of an unforgettable experience – that he was convinced should be part of dying. With permission, he began to walk around the local hospice, often stopping to talk to the patients, and to take the photos that they asked for; he provided a compassionate mirror in which they could see themselves for the last time.

In an article which he wrote about his experience, Murray gives an account of Wally, a dying man who troubled Murray because he sat with his wife, June, all day, and hardly spoke to her. Eventually, Murray stopped beside Wally's bed and on looking out of the window, he saw and photographed a magnificent rainbow. He showed it to Wally, saying lightly to him and June that a rainbow like that had to have a pot of gold at its end. At this, Wally finally began to talk. He told June that she was his pot of gold; he was not afraid to die, but found hope rising in his heart because he was so certain that she would join him when her time came. For her part, June seemed afloat with the joy that his words bestowed on her. Holding hands, they sat together for quite some time, at one in a blissful state. Wally died two days later, and although June wept, she still felt profoundly happy (Murray, 2015, p. 85).

Death of a young woman

Jane Zorza was only twenty-five when she developed an aggressive, malignant melanoma on her foot. Attractive to others, she was also a nonconformist, a questioner, impatient with banalities and superficialities, and someone who was not afraid of being different. As a teenager, she was prone to periods of depression and self-doubt; she liked to write poetry but being a perfectionist, she was seldom satisfied with what she had written. And now, in the midst of a life that was just beginning, she was confronted with the information that within months, it would come to a painful end. She was shocked and frightened.

In the event, Jane lived for only five more months, but there was one stroke of good fortune awaiting her. In 1967, the first hospice in the UK, St Christopher's, had opened its doors to offer palliative care to the dying. Others followed, and by 1977, when Jane Zorza most needed it, the Sir Michael Sobell House hospice offered a welcome to her, her family, and her many friends. Her parents, Victor and Rosemary Zorza, spent her last days with her, taking turns to sleep in a cot in her room. A former lover, Michael, came to see her, and they were able to resolve their unfinished business and say goodbye. By now, her pain was largely controlled, but she was losing her sight and her strength; however, she could still smell the rose left on her pillow each day, and use her hands to stroke the square of velvet she had asked for as a last special gift. Still able to hear, she could talk to her father about important, but hitherto unanswered questions that she had for him about his desperate life as a Polish Jew fleeing persecution and death in Eastern Europe during the Second World War. Rather more gently, she could allow herself to be bathed in her favourite music, Mozart's string quartets.

Near the end, Jane asked her mother to lie down with her – not a command, but a humble request – and with great difficulty, she moved her limp body closer to her mother; then, with a weak and awkward attempt to hold her mother in her arms, and with infinite tenderness, she said: "I do love you, Mum". At that, all the heartbreaks and strain of their lives together were put aside and forgiven.

On Jane's last day, with her body lying as if already dead, her breathing changed to a high and thin note, sounding deeply sad and distant. Then, it became so soft and light that her mother knew her time had come, and called her father: they took up their places on either side of Jane, each holding one of her hands. Her eyes opened a little for a second and then, everything about her became quite still. Ending their account of her death, Rosemary and Victor wrote:

> For us, who watched Jane's quiet end, there is a memory of her still, peaceful face and the warmth of her skin beneath our lips as we kissed her goodbye. This slow, gentle death was a natural end to life. The waning of her body was easy to believe and to accept. Her retreat had been strangely beautiful to watch. We felt no fear.
>
> (Zorza & Zorza, 1980, p. 249)

For those faced with dying alone

Death doula as companion to the dying

According to a study by anthropologist James Green, having someone with whom there is reciprocal love to sit with one at the last is the best way of all to die (Green, 2008, p. 18). For some, however, this will not be possible, and they face dying alone. But something of a remedy for this tragic lack has recently been initiated; there are trained individuals who can come to the rescue. They are called death doulas.

Jaki Fisher is a qualified death doula, someone who gives support to the dying; when invited, she sits with people who have no one else to be with them, and helps them in any way that she can. Jenny, a single woman dying in a hospice in Singapore, was Jaki's first client. Jenny was clear about what she wanted of Jaki; she had not really accepted dying and feared it, and she was anxious to avoid being left to die alone. Jaki undertook to stay with Jenny until she died, unless medical interventions prevented it. As Jenny got weaker, Jaki noticed something shift in her; Jenny told her that she was coming to accept what was happening.

At this point, Jenny began to tell Jaki how she wanted to pass her final days. Unable to eat, she wanted to see if she could maybe enjoy her beloved coffee again; when Jaki gave it to her, Jenny's eyes lit up with delight. She loved to be wheeled into the garden, where she would marvel at the simple joys of the birdsong, the flowers, and the sun and the wind. Not long after this, she deteriorated rapidly and died; Jaki was with her (Fisher, 2016).

The program responsible for this work is called the No One Should Die Alone Foundation (NOSDAF). For people who are dying alone, the NOSDAF volunteers become a virtual family, there just for them, right through to their last moment.

The future of ars moriendi

Whether occurring in a domestic or an institutional environment, each of these five vignettes demonstrates a configuration which respects the dying person's dignity and individuality, and reflects their cultural environment. It allows the love of friends and family for the dying person to be expressed up to their last moment; it also recognises that for people facing death alone, finding the right kind of companion can offer solace.

It has often been observed in this study that it is of great benefit to the dying to have some control over the way they experience their last days or weeks, and as Bourgeois and Johnson note, creating an *ars moriendi* is empowering to everyone involved (Bourgeois & Johnson, 2004, p. 105). Perhaps initiating the process earlier than might otherwise happen, professionals participating in the care of the dying can facilitate meaningful practices of this kind, and in so doing, they may enhance the individual's capacity not only to plan for their death but also, to come to accept it with grace.

Given that such deeply felt *ars moriendi* have so much meaning for the dying and for their friends and family, they may be capable of replacing the rituals for honouring the passing of loved ones that have been lost to our secular society.

Part IV. Limitations of the investigation, and areas for further research

Limitations of the investigation

Firstly, as a qualitative study with only five participants and the researcher making six, this is a small study and therefore, it is not generalisable. Where there are areas of agreement amongst the participants, however, it is possible that a wider trend might be indicated which could bear further investigation; an example of this would be participant endorsement of the need for creative disregard and another, that there may be a link between death awareness and retirement rather than literal age, with implications for programs like Advance Care Planning. There are also other findings which, though not agreed by all participants and perhaps, even applying only to one or two, are likely to produce working results and therefore, deserve further investigation. One such finding would be the possibility that radical disbelief is being confused with denial.

Secondly, the participants were all members of the middle class; working class attitudes to death and dying might be different in certain areas, though not necessarily in all. For example, working class people's ways of understanding what death is, and how to prepare for it, might not be the same as those of the present participants; being more generic, however, the form taken by the process of acceptance is likely to be widespread.

An obvious feature about the study is that the participants were all Caucasian, and people of other ethnicities, religions and cultural backgrounds were not included; they would each merit a study of their own. Other cultures may well differ radically, for example, in their ways of interpreting the meaning of death and its implications, and therefore, of preparing for it.

It should also be acknowledged that there was a further refinement of the selection of the participant group due to the choice of memoirs as data; all of the participants were educated, articulate and accomplished writers. However, this does not necessarily set them apart in attitudes from other middle-class Caucasians, rather, it may simply render them better able to communicate them. Further, the male participants were all eminent people with influence and prestige. However, having terminal cancer is a great leveller, and apart from the possible exception of the quality of the treatment they received, it is unlikely that the findings have been much affected by this circumstance.

Finally, on balance, it was thought to be most productive to focus the research on memoirs written by people actually facing death in the comparatively near future. However, given that they were typically recorded sometime after the participants had had the relevant thoughts, the use of written records as data rather than interviews might have reduced the immediacy of some of the material. Arguably, though, this does not necessarily imply that the memoirs were ultimately less truthful.

Areas for further research

The present study suggests the need for further research in a number of areas. Firstly, it is possible that, due to the untimeliness of their deaths, a group of participants who were at death a generation or more younger than those in the present study may well face a quite different trajectory in their dying.

Secondly, again for comparative purposes as well as for its intrinsic interest, research into the attitudes of people dying of diseases other than cancer would be rewarding. For example, although acceptance of death would probably follow a pattern similar to that of cancer sufferers, the experience of patients dying of neurological conditions like Motor Neurone disease or Multiple Sclerosis, or of heart and arterial disease or strokes, would be likely to raise their own issues, especially in regard to matters of care and support.

Of course, a study of the attitudes of working class people to their own death and dying is needed; the picture is incomplete without it. Further, in our multi-cultural society, a study is needed to investigate cultural differences in attitudes to death and dying between our Caucasian population, and large minority groups like our Chinese, Vietnamese and Indian compatriots.

As foreshadowed in the present study, a qualitative investigation of how religious people face death in comparison with the non-religious would be worthwhile and perhaps, might even yield some surprising results. Data from the present study suggests that there may be some so far hidden, but significant, changes in our secular society's attitudes to death that have negatively impacted our experience of dying in ways of which we are as yet unaware. Of course, the loss of hope of being received by a divine being and of the expectation of an afterlife, are often mentioned as significant casualties of our secularity; almost certainly, however, patterns of belief about the meaning of death and how it should be prepared for – while largely unconscious – have already begun to replace them. Arguably, it is time to study and document those schemata which are in process of forming, and those which are already in place.

As a companion piece to the present study, it would be interesting to carry out a study based on interviews with people of a similar age who, though not yet diagnosed as dying, would be willing to talk about their attitudes to the *prospect* of death and dying; its findings could then be compared with the accounts recorded by the dying in the present investigation.

Summary of chapters on research findings

Chapters 5–7, *Reaction to the news: Diagnosis, Living with dying,* and *Acceptance*, recounted the participants' journey from diagnosis to near-death. To carry the participants' narratives forward, and to identify which experiences were held in common and which were more individually held, a chronological presentation of the data was most effective.

This fourth and final chapter of research analysis has been presented in four parts. Part I explored the data which, taken together, provide an answer to the first 'burning question': *What is it like to face death?* Part II investigated the information gathered in response to the second burning question: *How can we become ready to relinquish life and accept death?* Part III supplied examples of *ars moriendi*, the art of dying well, while Part IV discussed the limitations of the study, and suggested further research which would build on the present investigation, and place it in a wider perspective.

References

Ballatt, J., & Campling, P. (2011). *Intelligent kindness: Reforming the culture of healthcare*. London: RCPsych Publications.

Bourgeois, S., & Johnson, A. (2004). Preparing for dying: Meaningful practices in palliative care. *Omega, 49*(2), 99–107. doi: 10.2190/1QQD-KVHM-FUD1-5V1M

Breitbart, W., Rosenfeld, B., Gibson, C., Pessin, H., Poppito, S., Nelson, C., … & Olden, C. (2010). Meaning-centred group psychotherapy for patients with advanced cancer: A pilot randomized controlled trial. *Psychooncology, 19*(1), 21–28. doi: 10.1002/pon.1556

Campbell, S. (2015, February 10). Atul Gawande's 5 questions to ask at life's end. *Next Avenue Newsletter for over 50's*. Retrieved from https://www.nextavenue.org/atul-gawandes-5-questions-ask-life's-end/

Carr, E. R. (2008). Quality of life for our patients: How media images and messages influence their perceptions. *Clinical Journal of Oncology Nursing, 12*(1), 43–51. doi:10.1188/08.CJON.43–51

Clarke, L. H., Korotchenko, A., & Bundon, A. (2012). 'The calendar is just about up': Older adults with multiple chronic conditions reflect on death and dying. *Ageing and Society, 32*(8), 1399–1417. Retrieved from https://www.ncbi.nlm.nih.gov/pubmed/24976657

Corke, C., & Hillman, K. (2018, July 28). *How to achieve a good death* [Interview with Geraldine Doogue, Radio National Saturday Extra]. Retrieved from http://www.abc.net.au/radionational/programs/saturdayextra/what-is-a-good-death/1C

Elias, N. (1985). *The loneliness of the dying*. E. Jephcott (Trans.). Oxford: Basil Blackwell Ltd.

Fisher, J. (2016, June 18). Becoming a 'death doula': Why I choose to sit with people as they die. *News.Com.Au.Real Life True Stories*. Retrieved from http://www.news.com.au/lifestyle/real-life/true-stories/becoming-a-death-doula-why-i-choose-to-sit-with-people-as-they-die/news-story/10273133ec193861c6b1b9d72a4630aa

Froggatt, K. (2001). Life and death in English nursing homes: Sequestration or transition? *Ageing and Society, 21*, 319–332. doi: 10.1017/S0144686X0100825X

Green, J. W. (2008). *Beyond the good death: The anthropology of modern dying*. Philadelphia: University of Pennsylvania Press.

Gum, A., & Snyder, C. R. (2002). Coping with terminal illness: The role of hopeful thinking. *Journal of Palliative Medicine, 5*(6), 883–894. Retrieved from https://www.ncbi.nlm.nih.gov/pubmed/12685535

Kuhl, D. (2003). *What dying people want: Practical wisdom for the end of life*. (1st ed.). New York: PublicAffairs.

McDermott, F., Hill, C., & Morgan, A. (2009). Death and the dynamics of group life. *Group Analysis, 42*(2), 156–176. doi: 10.1177/0533316409104363

Murray, T. (2015, August 25). Screen rites: Getting close to death and dying. *Humanities Australia,* 6, 82–91. Retrieved from http://find.lib.uts.edu.au/;jsessionid=64562982B89B4DD34E8A4CF8DEC755C2?R=OPAC_b2851249

Neimeyer, R. A., Wittkowski, J., & Moser, R. P. (2004). Psychological research on death attitudes. *Death Studies, 28*(4), 309–340. doi. 10.1080/07481180490432324

O'Reilly, M. (2014, September 25). "*Am I dying*?" [YouTube broadcast]. Retrieved from https://www.ted.com/talks/matthew_o_reilly_am_i_dying_the_honest_answer?language=en

Parkes, C., Relf, M., & Couldrick, A. (1996). *Counselling in terminal care and bereavement.* Baltimore, MD: Paul H. Brookes Publishing Co.

Patrick, D. L., Engelberg, R. A., & Curtis, J. S. (2001). Evaluating the quality of dying and death. *Journal of Pain and Symptom Management, 22*(3), 717–726. https://www.jpsmjournal.com/

Price, K., & Cheek, J. (2007). Avoiding death: The ultimate challenge in the provision of contemporary healthcare? *Health Sociology Review, 16*(5), 397–404. doi: 10.5172/hesr.2007.16.5.397

Schroepfer, T. A., Noh, H., & Kavanaugh, M. (2009). The myriad strategies for seeking control in the dying process. *The Gerontologist, 49*(6), 755–766. doi: 10.1093/geront/gnp060

Sullivan, M. D. (2003). Hope and hopelessness at the end of life. *The American Journal of Geriatric Psychiatry, 11*(4), 393–405. Home page URL: https://www.ajgponline.org/

Stanley, L., & Wise, S. (2011). The domestication of death: The sequestration thesis and domestic figuration. *Sociology, 45*(6), 947–962. doi: 10.1177/0038038511416153

Zorza, R., & Zorza, V. (1980). *A way to die: Living to the end.* New York: Knopf.

9 Conclusions

Introduction

Research into how we face death is a late arrival in the thanatological literature. According to Stanley and Wise (2011, p. 950), as recently as the 1990s, even a respected sociologist like Anthony Giddens was still writing about the human attitude to personal death as if everyone dealt with it in the same way. More than a decade later, physician and academic, Michael Bartalos, expressed concern about the continuing lack of studies of "patients facing death but not yet dying", with the capacity during that time to be aware of, and to reflect on their experience (2009, p. 232). Like Kubler-Ross, Bartalos was in favour of terminal patients being encouraged to reflect on their experience of the finiteness of life, and he deprecated the fact that this had not happened – neither in our institutions, nor in everyday thinking. As a consequence, in Bartalos' view, our notions of the subjective experience of facing death have remained theoretical and academic. Indeed, as far as is known to the author, until the present study was undertaken, the gap in our knowledge of what it is like for someone to face death over months, or even years, has remained unfilled. As a first step in remedying this lack, Chapter 8, *Themes in the experience of dying*, has shown that, *en route* to providing the answers to the questions asked in Chapter 1, this modest investigation has produced enough data to furnish thirty-two wide-ranging themes across eleven clusters.

This final chapter first draws on the data analysis narratives and the findings of Chapter 8 to furnish answers to the questions set out in Chapter 1. Some observations on the unique problems of thinking about one's own death follow, leading to a discussion of why it has been impossible until recently to research the subjective experience of facing death and dying. Some reflections on the timeliness of this enquiry, and the likelihood of there being more such explorations to come, bring the chapter, and the book, to a close.

Response to Question 1

The first question in the investigation asks: *What is it like to face death?* A full answer to this question is descriptive, but complex; it has to address the

DOI: 10.4324/9781003392088-9

physical, emotional and psychological domains of the study group participants' experience, from diagnosis to death.

One of the greatest demands on the participants was to persevere with everyday life in the face of the suffering caused by the illness and its treatment. Despite advances in modern medicine, most terminal diseases are harrowing to those who suffer them, and patients can take a long time to die. Periods of reflection on life and death are regularly swept aside by the progress of disabling symptoms on the one hand, and their treatment regimens on the other. In this case, where cancer was the shared affliction, as well as suffering from their particular form of the disease, all participants had to bear the side effects of heavy-duty chemotherapy and radiation therapy. In addition, Gould had two major surgical interventions, and Mayne and Taylor, one; Diski and Hitchens both had inoperable tumours. Since no participant's experience of dying was the same as any of the others, each must be described individually.

As a result of the damage done to her lungs by radiotherapy designed to shrink her inoperable tumour, Diski's pulmonary fibrosis became terminal, exposing her to regular bouts of near-suffocation controlled only by orally administered morphine, and the use of a hand-held, battery-powered electric fan. Notably hard on cancer patients, her chemotherapy rendered her too fatigued to stay awake for more than a few hours a day, caused frequent vomiting, made most food unappetising or inedible, and caused her slight frame to become bloated. Having become terminally ill with both lung cancer and pulmonary fibrosis, Diski described herself as haunted by a former GP exclaiming: "Oh Jenny, they're both such terrible ways to die" (Diski, p. 166).

Diagnosed with a non-metastasised large tumour of the oesophagus close to his stomach, Gould was first offered surgery which would have involved breaking his ribs, and entering his stomach and upper chest by major incision. Unable at this stage to accept this, he and his wife accepted a less radical, alternative surgery confined to his stomach. As it turned out, it was possible that the cancer later became terminal because Gould's chosen first surgery was insufficiently radical, and failed to remove all of the cancer; a second surgery to correct this was ineffective. After both surgeries, his pain was for some time impossible to control. Following large amounts of chemotherapy and radiation therapy, he could not eat during his last months, and was fed through a tube inserted in his stomach. Emaciated by then, he died in ICU from an overwhelming lung infection.

Having taken a combative stand towards his stage four inoperable oesophageal cancer, Hitchens accepted massive doses of chemotherapy and radiotherapy. Thus, until he died from an untreatable lung infection contracted in the hospital, his main struggle was with the side effects of his treatment. His voice became a piping squeak, and his hands, as he put it, were threatening to become dead; he described the loss of these functions – essential to a public intellectual – as threatening to annihilate his very personality and identity. Seemingly well-grounded, he in fact suffered agonies from a traumatised imagination. For example, having investigated, experienced and suffered post-traumatic stress disorder from the effects of water-boarding, he sometimes felt rising panic when washed by nurses; further, chemotherapy confused him, and left him fearful that his mind might become so addled by it that he would mistake treatment for torture, an overture to a gruesome execution.

Like Gould, Mayne underwent surgery soon after diagnosis, and spent twelve hours in theatre. Several parts of his mouth and neck were removed to excise the cancer and then, reconstructed from flesh from his thigh. After the surgery, he experienced uncontrollable pain and terrifying hallucinations from the drugs he was given, and found it difficult to sustain feeling in touch with God. He had lost his teeth, and found speaking and eating painfully taxing. Then, not long after the surgery, he was told that some small cancers had been missed. Accordingly, he underwent radiotherapy – which attacked his ruined mouth cruelly – only to be told later by a new consultant that it had probably not been necessary. Not long after being discharged as cured, he became ill again, and was given a terminal diagnosis. Despite having malodorous open cancer sores in this throat, he spent his last weeks without further treatment, in order to retain as much quality of life as possible.

Less is known about the progress of Taylor's stage four melanoma and its treatment because much of it occurred in the nine years before she began the memoir. Since she was able to continue writing and keep her condition secret even from her adult sons during that time, it may, in its early stages, have been rather less distressing than was the case for the other four participants. She did not begin the memoir until nine years post-onset, shortly after having surgery for seizures caused by metastases in her brain; her prognosis by then was about a year. As a result of the surgical intervention, she suffered a loss of the motor functions needed for driving and walking and, unable to eat much, she gradually became frail and weak, developing a number of protruding tumours; finally, she drifted into a comatose state, and died.

It might be imagined that the physical aspect of facing death by cancer would have been so debilitating and preoccupying that, however much some relief from it might have been longed for, the participants would not have had the strength or the spirit to engage in anything beyond bare survival. While for some individuals that might be the case, it is not inevitable. In fact, living and dying take place alongside one another for a time, until the living gradually comes to a halt, and the dying goes full term. Accordingly, it might then be thought that if this is the case, living must surely be a poor and increasingly jaded or perhaps, an ever more desperate and intense affair. It is true that the dying have to accept arduous burdens and strains daily that are not encountered by well persons, but the quality of the inner lives of the individuals in this study shows that even in extremis, at life's end, human beings can find resources within themselves that they would not have believed could exist. Accordingly, the next two sections relate to the emotional and psychological aspects of the participants' dying.

……

While the physical suffering was immense, managing their emotional and psychological issues was at least equally demanding on the study's participants. Facing death was for all of them, a time of intense distress and anxiety, and although they were all well supported by their families and friends, their resources were regularly stretched to the limit.

A metaphor for a hard death, often preceded by a cruel illness and a harsh treatment regimen, all the participants found dying from cancer *per se* stressful. No doubt other diseases – neurological conditions like motor neurone disease, for example – would, in their own way, be similarly stressful. Alongside the cloud cast on them by the cancer's inimical presence, lay the prospect of parting forever from their spouses and families, a tragedy which, despite their becoming accustomed to it to some degree, could hang over them for months, or even years. Further, over time, they would have to accept the loss of control of almost everything that was important to them, which was seldom accompanied by an equivalent loss of the desire to manage their own lives. Finally, difficult as it was within the medical systems they needed to inhabit, it was essential to all the participants to maintain their individuality; intent upon avoiding the fate of becoming 'unpersons' – 'the terminally-ill', or 'an advanced cancer patient' – they were all determined to remain, and to be recognised as their authentic selves to the end.

At this time of final goodbyes, there were three participants who, deserted by their parents as children, experienced a reactivation of their fears of abandonment, a fear that their again being helpless and in need might cause the vital link between them and those who represented their security to break down. One participant, Diski, could not find a stable sense of security in the reassurances from her family that they were there for her, but Mayne and Taylor did recover their confidence that, as well as their devoted families, they were loved by those whom they revered – he, by his God, and she, by her mother.

In order to endure their ordeal, all participants found their own way to counteract its rigours; for one participant, this involved the use of mood-changing ploys, for another, having a euthanising drug to hand in case the suffering became too great; for the men in particular, it was shutting down negative thoughts like self-pity, which might otherwise have undermined their inner strength. For four of them, having a dependable means of control over being engulfed in unbearable thoughts and feelings, allowed them to retain some sense of still being in charge of themselves; in Diski's case, however, her attempts to remain in control were continually under threat. Finally, all participants found and relied upon outside support to accompany them during the long haul – partners, family, friends, medical professionals, religious individuals and communities, groups such as Exit International, and counselling.

For four of the participants, their resourcefulness paid dividends, and they were freed to spend time writing and thinking; the fifth, Diski, could find no reliable way of managing her anxieties, and although she continued writing her memoir for some time, she gradually became swamped by them.

……

For all participants, there were hazardous times of psychological upheaval, all of which required arduous periods of working through the associated psychological issues; throughout, there were episodes that were profoundly moving.

As described in Chapter 7, *Resolution of conflicts* and *Confessions*, all participants endured anguish over conflicts which had gnawed at them below the surface of their minds for years, or even for a lifetime. As if aware that this was their last chance to be made right, still unresolved accounts of real or imagined damage done to, and by the participants besieged them, demanding to be resolved. As part of this work of resolution, Mayne experienced horrific accusatory hallucinations which brought him to his knees, Taylor considered suicide over her fears of becoming a helpless burden, Hitchens imagined screaming for a priest and dying by torture, Gould endured crushing guilt over failing his wife, and Diski obsessed over her rejection by Doris Lessing as though it were happening afresh every day.

One being the author, two participants received, but could not take in the diagnosis of terminal lung cancer, because they had no matching sense of impairment; that is, they were subject to radical disbelief. Given that the diagnosis was not in dispute, these participants experienced the same fears regarding imminent death as their peers; moreover, at times incorrectly assessed as being unco-operative or in denial, both felt isolated and silenced by the incomprehension and dismissiveness of medical professionals who were intolerant of what they took to be avoidance. For the author, recovery came with a correction of the misdiagnosis, and with understanding the experience and writing about it; however, although there was a touching moment when she imagined her beloved grandson sturdily dealing with her unhelpful oncologist, Diski sought, but was never helped, to connect with and accept her diagnosis. A similarly depersonalising event occurred when Diski received a prognosis based on statistical probability, rather than on a more individualised assessment of what quality and duration of life was left to her. The resultant undermining of her sense of the length and shape of her future left her feeling impotent, without agency, adding to her tendency to question what value she could attach to her life, or to herself.

Two participants withdrew from engagement with others; Diski became convinced that she could no longer trust the medical professionals around her, while Hitchens was determined to block any attempt to sympathise with how he felt about his illness and oncoming death. Although Hitchens probably knew his own limits best, had Diski's oncologist been familiar with the work of Colin Parkes (1996) and his team, she might have experienced feeling better understood and hence, more secure; given the dynamic activity in the psyche of those facing death, with a timely intervention from an experienced crisis counsellor, she might even have had her tragic end turned around. The other three participants remained engaged to the end.

On the other side of the ledger, no participant denied or faced away from their impending death and indeed, Taylor, Mayne and Gould all indicated that confronting death squarely led to their fear of it making way for good experiences. All participants could lose themselves in the activity of their writing, the enjoyment of their particular form of creative disregard. A rewarding and worthwhile way of spending the time they had left, their work also diverted their attention away from the illness, and prevented the development of an obsession with details of the effects of their treatment, or the evidence of their decline. For those participants with a capacity for objective self-analysis – for example, Gould, Mayne and Taylor – what they experienced and recorded expressed a flowering of their insight into themselves and the world around them. Reaching into depths that they had never before been able to plumb, they forgave betrayals that they had not, until this point, felt able to forgive, and acknowledged sins of their own for which they needed to be forgiven. Although their sadness remained, for these three participants, dying was also a time of intense, at times transcendent experience, and unique insight. Of the other two, Hitchens remained sturdily true to himself, but Diski finally broke down into incoherence.

In the final analysis, no participant suffered to a degree that was beyond their capacity to contain, reflect on and in some form, survive; Mayne became resolute and master of his fate, Gould experienced a quasi-mystical love for all creation, Taylor drifted into an oceanic state of union with all things, Hitchens acknowledged that is was his mortality that entitled him to freedom of thought and expression, and although she had a possibly self-protective breakdown, Diski arguably underwent a kind of redemption.

Response to Question 2

The second question in the investigation asks: *If our most basic instinct is to survive, how can we become ready to relinquish life and accept death?* This question represents a challenge to a commonly-held theory about human functioning – our belief in the existence of a 'survival instinct' – requiring an observational-analytical answer which, if inconsistent with it, could bring the universal applicability of that theory into question.

To progress the investigation of this issue, the question must first be asked: what is involved in the acceptance of death, and how is it accessed?

Firstly, the research reveals that for those four of the five participants who were able to accept death, it seemed to be a state of being rather than the gift of an article of faith or the outcome of reasoning, the result of being able to access the inscription that like birth, dying is an inevitable and natural event, a process of letting go which requires no specialised know-how.

Secondly, the research finds that it is not so much that the instinct to survive and acceptance of dying are opposites or alternatives, in which the existence of one state disproves or brings into the question the existence of the other. Rather, both states are inscriptions in our genetic endowment, and both are present throughout our lives. In the midst of life, the survival instinct is typically the predominant presence in the awareness of psychologically well individuals, while the potential to respond to being faced with death is repressed. However, when the individual realises that dying in the foreseeable future has become part of his reality, the disposition towards accepting death will ordinarily be activated; both states will thereafter co-exist simultaneously for the rest of his or her life. A dying man will typically leap out of the path of an oncoming bus.

A footnote is needed here: Acceptance of death must be distinguished from *resignation* to it; in the process of *accepting* it, death is recognised as the fitting endpoint of the lived experience of one's life, while being *resigned* to death involves putting up with, or enduring it, as something highly unpleasant, even intolerable, because there is no way of preventing or escaping it.

While the inscription in our genetic endowment that governs accepting death is universal, there may be barriers to our being able to access it.

The nature of Diski's inability to accept death was spelt out in her conviction that she could not 'do' dying. In her imagination, dying involved being hurled in a lone dive into the cosmos, followed by a collapse into meltdown; worst of all, she expected to remain conscious throughout until finally being forever exiled, presumably to nowhere.

There are two aspects to the process of losing the knowledge that dying is natural, and that one can allow oneself to let go and drift into eternity. Firstly, due to its having been overwritten by a different and potent inscription, which suppresses it, access to the relevant inscription has been lost. In Diski's case – originally intended to ensure her survival – the overwritten inscription might have been something like: 'Never surrender'. In order for the original inscription to be restored, resolution of a relevant, usually central and persistent conflict which would simultaneously remove the overwritten inscription, would be required. Unfortunately, Diski's inability to resolve her problems with the Lessings and achieve the peace of mind needed to access acceptance of death was governed by the same inscription: 'Never surrender', as her confession made clear. As long as she could not give up basing her relationships largely on satirical distancing or covert war, and acknowledge her need for giving and receiving love without reservation, she would remain governed by: 'Never surrender'. Arguably, however, although the overwritten inscription remained in place, her tenderness for her grandchildren had swept Diski up into a state of unconditional love alongside, and creating a powerful exception to it. While she never retrieved a loving internal parent for her cruelly abused young self in the way that Mayne and Taylor had done, Diski's recovery of a motherly presence may still have occurred, but in a different way. Perhaps her final thoughts can be understood as the make-believe chatter of an imaginative little girl to a make-believe mother with whom, hand-in-hand, she is going home.

Secondly, Diski's fantasy about her final terrifying swan dive into nowhere illustrates a further barrier to accepting dying; it conflates dying with being killed, which must surely preclude acceptance. For those who cannot accept that dying is natural, dying and being killed have probably become merged. Hitchens was another near-victim of this category error; believing for some time that he might experience it as an execution, he had remained determined to fight death off. Shortly before he rather unexpectedly died, however, he had apparently been enlightened by Lightman's credo that immortality would make us all prisoners of ancestral tyranny; at that point, he seems to have become persuaded that preserving freedom of thought was worth dying for. Now, as Kubler-Ross originally believed that the human unconscious did not accept that life could end, she had formed the view that every human being must unconsciously believe that death meant being killed as a punishment for doing something wicked. In fact, rather than confirming this hypothesis, the present research shows that it represents an aberration of the normal process of acceptance. Indeed, being able to access the disposition to accept dying is conditional upon the individual's capacity to exclude the belief that dying is the equivalent of being killed.

A cautionary note may be appropriate here. It is to be hoped that our seemingly ever-increasing reluctance to access the inscription for acceptance of death as natural will not mean that eventually, it will become unavailable to us. If, as a society, we were to succeed in permanently repressing the inscription, death acceptance would be replaced by the widespread expectation that we will – indeed, must – never die. It would be hard to overstate the catastrophic effects of such a development; certainly, there would be far too many of us battling for far too few of the necessities of life. As things stand at present, however, the acceptance of dying is still inscribed within us and once known, when death is imminent, it emerges as an unequivocal state of affairs which will unfold in its own way.

……

In conclusion, given that we cannot give an account of our own deaths because death wipes out the first-person witness position, according to Secomb (2002), the nearest alternative is to write about "being-towards-death" (p. 33). As Secomb observes, both death- and survival-seeking are fundamental to our instinctual endowment, a view that was first put forward by Freud in 1920. Nowadays, it is widely agreed that when we face impending death, our task in thinking about it is not so much to construct a challenging new scenario, as to undo or bypass the repression which, as Freud (1920) claimed, had until then prevented us from accessing what we have always known. Of course, for most people, lifting a lifelong repression of the path to death and finding the way to acceptance involves time, and often, great turmoil. Accordingly, would-be researchers into the subjective experience of dying would expect to encounter major, perhaps insuperable difficulties in enrolling individuals facing death in longitudinal research programs. The Death Zone, as Gould called it, is a profoundly private domain; permission to enter it for persons other than family and friends, and medical or other relevant personnel, is not readily available. Indeed, there seems little doubt that the absence until now of research into the experience of dying is the result of these very problems.

However, there has been a development in recent years which has made such research far more practicable. Although autothanatography has existed since the Middle Ages, writing for the general public about one's own death has really flourished in the last few decades; access to memoirs of the dying has made longitudinal research into facing our own death possible at last. But why has writing memoirs about one's own dying become so popular? In our secular society, which is so lacking in widely-accepted belief frameworks for the dying, perhaps it is a sign, as Stanley and Wise (2011) have it, that we want to draw in, and make ineffable death part of our everyday understanding of our world, to allow us to ready ourselves for when it is our time to die. Further research in this field seems certain to follow.

References

Bartalos, M. (2008). *Speaking of death: America's new sense of mortality.* Westport, CT: Praeger Publishers.

Freud, S. (1920/1987 version). *On Metapsychology: Beyond the pleasure principle.* Harmondsworth, Middlesex: Penguin Books.

Kubler-Ross, E. (1969). *Death and dying.* New York: Macmillan Publishing Company.

Parkes, C., Relf, M., & Couldrick, A. (1996). *Counselling in terminal care and bereavement.* Baltimore, MD: Paul H. Brookes Publishing Co.

Secomb, L. (2002). Autothanatography. *Mortality,* 7(1), 33–46. doi: 10.1080/13576270120102535

Stanley, L., & Wise, S. (2011). The domestication of death: The sequestration thesis and domestic figuration. *Sociology, 45*(6), 947–962. doi: 10.1177/0038038511416153

Index

For Product Safety Concerns and Information please contact our EU representative GPSR@taylorandfrancis.com Taylor & Francis Verlag GmbH, Kaufingerstraße 24, 80331 München, Germany